Surgical Anatomy
AROUND the ORBIT
The System of Zones

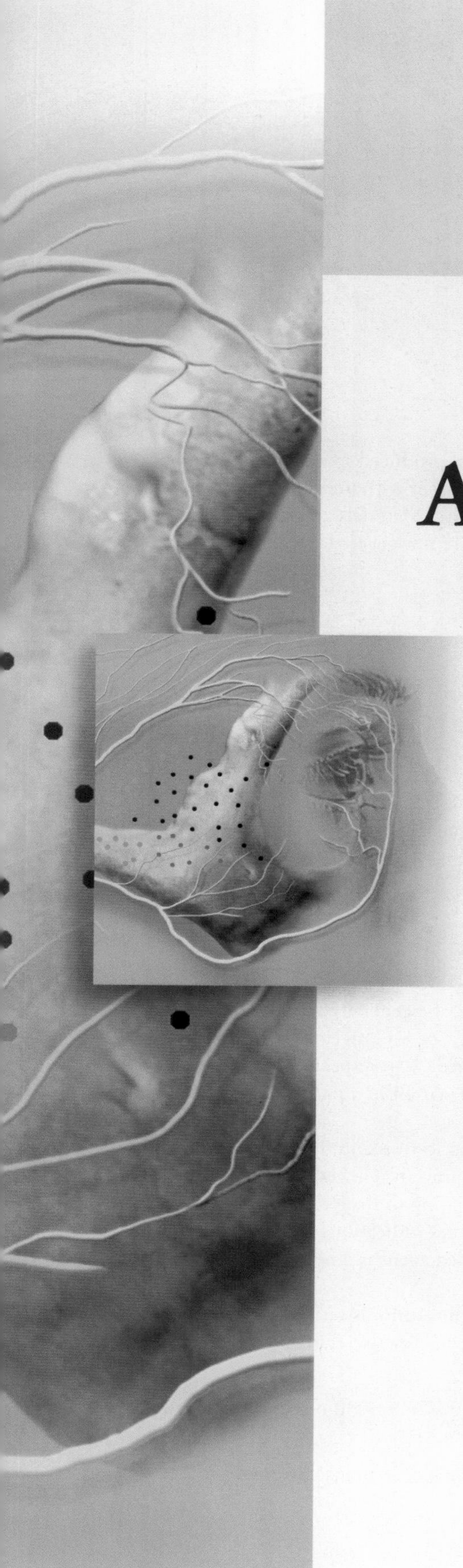

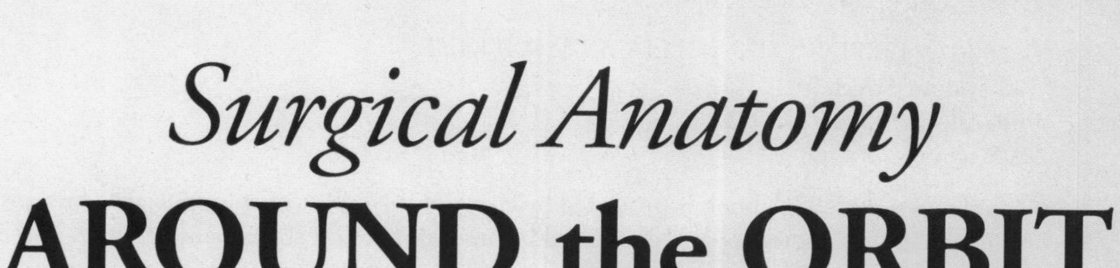

Surgical Anatomy AROUND the ORBIT

The System of Zones

BARRY M. ZIDE, M.D., D.M.D.
Professor of Surgery (Plastic)
Institute of Reconstructive Surgery
New York University Medical Center
New York, New York

ILLUSTRATOR: Craig A. Luce, M.S.

ASSOCIATE PROSECTORS:
SEAN BOUTROS, M.D., skilled surgeon and one of NYU's finest residents and recent graduates, and
ARTHUR MILLMAN, M.D., close friend and confidant, brilliant ophthalmic surgeon, and very clear thinker.

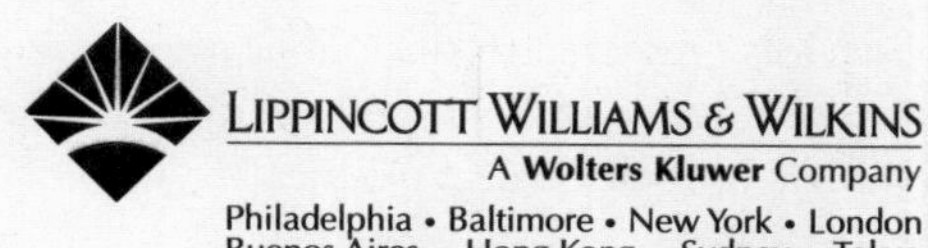

LIPPINCOTT WILLIAMS & WILKINS
A Wolters Kluwer Company
Philadelphia • Baltimore • New York • London
Buenos Aires • Hong Kong • Sydney • Tokyo

Acquisitions Editor: Jonathan Pine
Developmental Editor: Jenny Kim
Project Manager: Fran Gunning
Manufacturing Manager: Ben Rivera
Marketing Manager: Adam Glazer
Creative Director: Doug Smock
Cover and Interior Design: Karen Kappe
Production Services: Nesbitt Graphics, Inc.
Printer: Quebecor World-Kingsport

530 Walnut Street
Philadelphia, PA 19106 USA
LWW.com

Printed in the USA

A continuation of Zide & Jelks: Surgical Anatomy of the Orbit
Raven Press, 1985

Library of Congress Cataloging-in-Publication Data
Surgical anatomy around the orbit / editor, Barry M. Zide.
p. ; cm.
ISBN 0-7817-5081-4
1. Eye-sockets—Atlases. 2. Eye-sockets—Surgery—Atlases. I. Zide, Barry M. [DNLM:
1. Orbit—anatomy & histology—Atlases. 2. Orbit—surgery—Atlases. 3. Cranial Nerves—
Atlases. 4. Facial Bones—Atlases. 5. Ocular Physiology—Atlases. WW 17 S961 2006]
QM511.S875 2006
611'.84—dc22

2005007129

To purchase additional copies of this book, call our customer service department at (800) 639-3030 or fax orders to (301) 824-7390. International customers should call (301) 714-2324.

Visit Lippincott Williams & Wilkins on the Internet at LWW.com. Lippincott Williams & Wilkins customer service representatives are available from 8:30 am to 6 pm, EST.

10 9 8 7 6

Dedication

To my incredible summa wife, Linda, whose happy smile and kisses in the morning send me off with a great start every day. Am I lucky?!!

Special Acknowledgments

JOSEPH G. MCCARTHY, M.D., for his unbridled, unfailing enthusiasm toward this project, and

JONATHAN W. PINE JR., of Lippincott Williams & Wilkins, for making this work possible.

Preface

*Y*OU MIGHT BE ASKING, *What could possibly change about anatomy since 1985 when the first edition arrived?* ANSWER*—nothing. What has changed is what we surgeons are doing around the orbit and, because of that, a refocused upgrade was required.*

The development of endoscopic techniques, treatment of ptotic brow problems, the advanced methods of deep plane surgery and midface lifts meant that a more detailed study and presentation of the periocular anatomy was due. The concepts and words of "ROOF" (retro-orbicularis oculi fat), "SOOF" (suborbicularis oculi fat), the galeal fat pads, and cutaneous ligaments showed up; the nuances of such anatomy became somewhat mysterious because the presentations were befuddling. Certain retaining ligaments and septae required understanding. The anatomic concepts of fat repositioning and the anatomy relevant to approaches to perform certain maneuvers were not emphasized in the earlier edition. Finally, the seventh nerve has always been there, with studies galore to help the surgeon, but never combined to describe the exact zone of safety and what is really innervated. In addition, because the environs allow us to use the local nerve exits to block much of the face, the anatomy even for nerve blocks for the entire face are described in depth. Foolproof block techniques are provided.

Once again the dissections are very fresh, and the schematics show information added as required. Herein, you will see periorbital anatomy as you have never seen it before, in an understandable, exciting (I hope), readable way, all glorified by the magnificent artwork of Craig A. Luce, in my opinion the finest ophthalmic artist of our day. What better way to prepare for surgery could there be? As before, I beg the indulgence and forgiveness of many great surgeons, authors, and anatomists, whose data I have extracted without giving specific credit. There is no bibliography, yet exhaustive research was crucial for the substance of this volume. The new pictures are larger and the color truer, and each one only shows several key points at most. Any dissections that seemed distracting, e.g., poorly focused, erratically colored, or repetitious, were left out. Only the *best* dissections were savored to show true anatomical concepts. You all know, of course, that variations commonly exist and labels were reduced drastically to avoid clutter and to allow this book to be read easily from picture to picture. Very little overlap exists between the first volume except in the first chapter, and that has been upgraded and changed considerably because of recent advances.

Diligent surgeons like you always try to improve your results, always try to do new things, and always try to remain current. With these dissections, your horizons of understanding will expand. That remains my purpose and my promise.

Barry M. Zide, M.D., D.M.D.
Institute of Reconstructive Surgery
New York University Medical Center

Foreword

The tradition of anatomic studies in the development of modern medicine has a long and proud history. Herophilus (approximately 300 B.C.) was likely the first person to dissect both humans and animals for learning purposes. Galen (129–199 A.D.) continued this tradition with a 16-book treatise, *On Anatomical Procedure.* His anatomical studies, drawn mainly from animals, were inherited by Vesalius. As a student at the Universities of Louvain and Paris, Vesalius (born in Brussels, 1514), initiated the modern era of surgery with the publication of *Fabrica* in 1543 while a professor at Padua. For the first time surgery was placed on a sound anatomic basis. In *Fabrica* (book VII), he described the eye and orbit, however, with only minimal detail and a multitude of erroneous descriptions.

When I was a medical student in the 1960s, a perception existed that all that was to be known about human anatomy was already available in textbooks and, moreover, the subject had been totally exhausted by "19th-century German anatomists." This misconception was regrettably reflected in an erosion of time allocated for the study of anatomy by curriculum committees at all medical schools.

How ironic! If you look at recent developments in plastic surgery over the last fifty years, it is obvious that crucial anatomic studies, done by practicing plastic surgeons, propelled the discipline into the future.

Paul Tessier, as a young Parisian surgeon in the 1960s, spent weekends at his alma mater in Brittany doing detailed anatomic studies of the craniofacial region. This information provided the foundation for the new field of craniofacial surgery.

In like manner, a cadre of young American plastic surgeons (Arnold, McCraw, Bostwick, Mathes, Nahai) studied the vascular supply not only to the skin, but also to the underlying musculature. These studies presaged the development of a vibrant era of innovative flat surgery. These vascular anatomy studies followed a long tradition going back to the injection studies of the pioneering father of surgical research, John Hunter, in the late 18th century. Moreover, in the first half of the 20th century, Truetta and others had extended the technique to demonstrate the blood supply of bone.

The bottom line is the following: Surgeons have recognized the relevance of anatomic studies to advance their discipline, by designing new surgical techniques that are not only innovative, but also less invasive.

It is with this background that Dr. Zide, master plastic surgeon and anatomist, has gone back to the anatomy laboratory to provide more insight into the structures of the periorbital region, especially in their relationship to existing techniques. As a practicing surgeon, recognizing the limitations of the traditional anatomic concepts of this region, he began a modern anatomic odyssey, the fruits of which are so elegantly presented in this text. Using only fresh or semi-fresh specimens, the author has photographically documented the fine anatomic details of the periorbital region. The practicing surgeon, by examining the photographs and the correlative drawings and watercolor paintings of the talented artist, Craig A. Luce, can not only improve surgical technique but, more importantly, can in turn use the material to design new techniques to be added to the surgical armamentarium.

Dr. Zide has again demonstrated the rewards of anatomic studies conducted by a practicing surgeon. It is only the latter who truly appreciates the importance of a thorough understanding of the multiple layers of the orbital soft tissues, the bony configurations, and the interrelationships of the soft tissues and skeleton.

Here is a most rewarding text not only for the student, but also for the practicing surgeon, because all of us in surgery are students forever.

Joseph G. McCarthy, M.D.
Lawrence D. Bell Professor of Plastic Surgery
New York University School of Medicine
Director, Institute of Reconstructive Plastic Surgery
New York University Medical Center

Table of Contents

CHAPTER 1

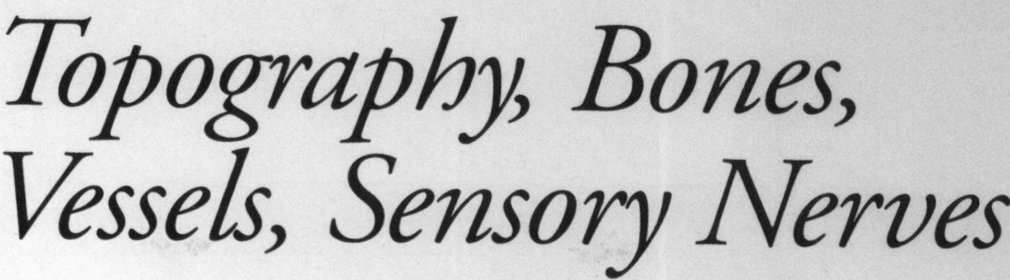

Topography, Bones, Vessels, Sensory Nerves

1 The ocular globes reside in two symmetrical bony cavities called the orbits.

2 Nerves and vessels enter the orbit, and their course and distribution must be understood. The aerated sinuses as well as the anterior and middle cranial fossae are intimately related to the orbital walls. The first edition, *Surgical Anatomy of the Orbit,* focused on this orbit and its contents, but very little on the neighboring areas. This edition expands widely, leaving the orbital confines to expose structures around it. Some basics are still required, so this initial chapter was rewritten to present an updated compendium of the essential data.

3 In this portion, you will learn certain orbital distances and relationships that you, the surgeon, will need to commit to memory. For that reason, some key numbers may be repeated.

Notes to the reader: *Throughout this book, all dissections use the right orbit. Labels are kept to a minimum so as not to distract the reader; perusing the legends will allow the pictures to really tell the story. This approximates "truth" where labels do not exist.*

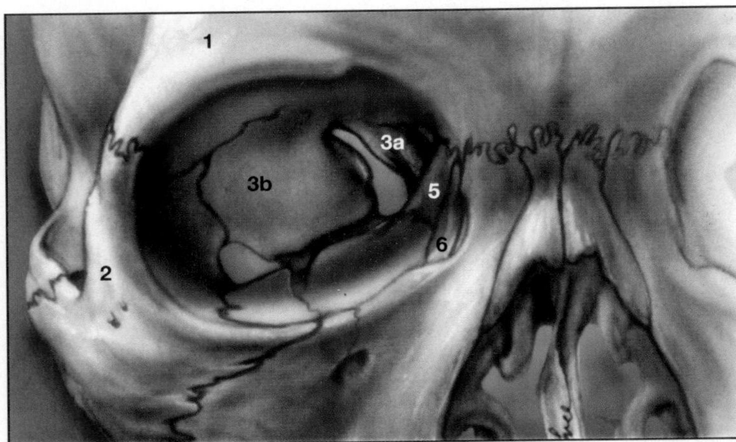

Figure 1.1A Bony components of the right orbit

1. Frontal bone (*orange*)
2. Zygoma (*light gray*)
3. Sphenoid bone (*purple*)

3a. Lesser wing

3b. Greater wing

Maxilla (*tan*)

Ethmoid bone (*purple* - *5*)

Lacrimal bone (*6*)

Palatine bone (no. 4 below)

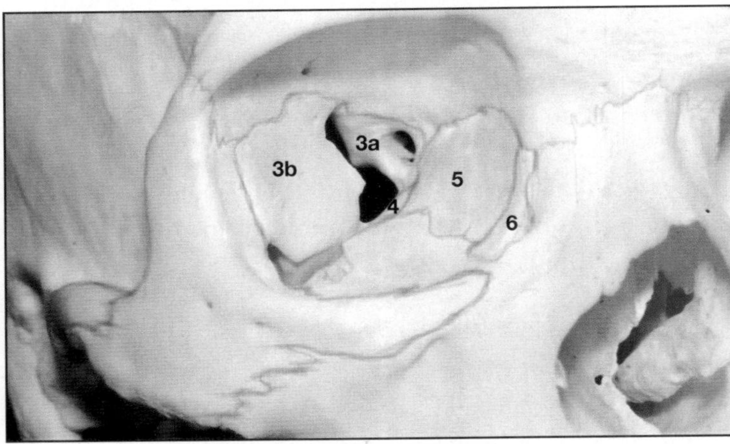

Figure 1.1B Dried skull with bony borders accented

3a. Lesser wing of sphenoid

3b. Greater wing sphenoid

4. Palatine bone
5. Ethmoid bone
6. Lacrimal bone

Figure 1.2 Anatomic points

1. The infraorbital foramen(*) opens downward and medially.
2. Red arrows point to exits of zygomaticofacial sensory nerve branches which supply the malar eminence and below.
3. The width of the lateral orbital rim inferior line is 1.3 to 1.5 cm.
4. The width of the lateral orbital rim at canthal level is 1.0 to 1.1 cm (*dotted*), and thinner as it approaches zygomatico-frontal suture (blue arrow).
5. Intraorbital arrows:
   Anterior and posterior ethmoidal foramina separate frontal bone above from ethmoid bone below it at the fronto-ethmoidal suture.

The anterior foramen is 20 mm behind the anterior orbital margin, and the posterior is 12 mm behind this. The ophthalmic artery gives off the posterior ethmoidal arteries for the posterior ethmoidal air cells, anterior cranial fossa dura, and upper nasal mucosa. The anterior ethmoidal artery enters the anterior cranial fossa, and then via the cribriform plate into the nose.

The anterior ethmoidal nerve, a sensory branch of the nasociliary, supplies anterior ethmoidal air cells, mucosa of the upper nose, and then exists as the dorsal nasal nerve (responsible for herpes zoster of the nasal tip).

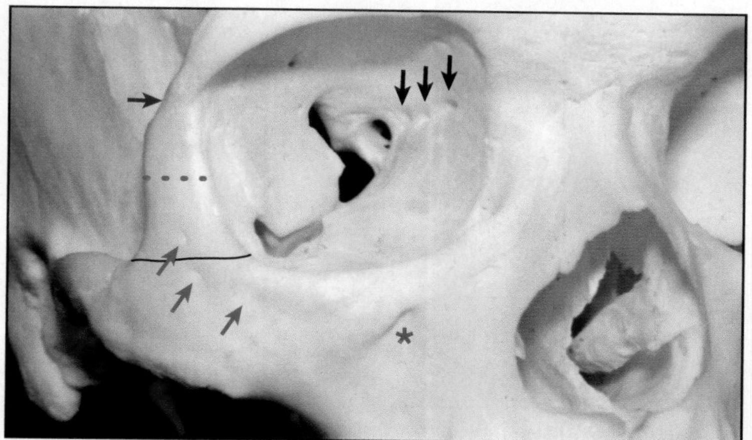

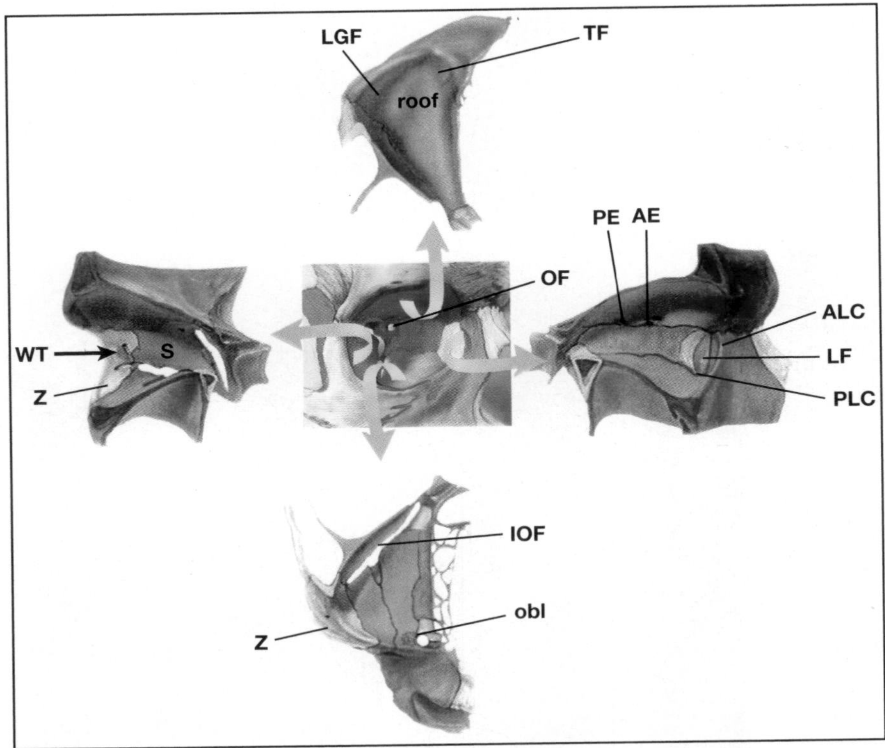

Figure 1.3 The walls

The roof. This wall is composed mainly of the orbital plate of the frontal bone. Posteriorly, it receives a minor contribution from the lesser wing of the sphenoid bone.

Located within the anterolateral portion of the roof, note a smooth, wide depression for the lacrimal gland, the lacrimal fossa (LGF). Approximately 5 mm posterior to the medial aspect of the rim, the trochlear fossa (TF) denotes the attachment of the cartilaginous pulley for the tendon of the superior oblique muscle. The triangular roof narrows as it proceeds toward the apex, where a vertically oval opening, the optic foramen (OF), marks the orbital end of the optic canal.

The lateral wall. The lateral wall is formed primarily by the orbital surface of the zygomatic bone (Z) and the greater wing of the sphenoid bone (S).

A small, bony promontory may be noted just within the orbital rim. This important landmark, Whitnall's tubercle (WT), is the point of attachment for several structures 11 mm below the zygomaticofrontal suture. At the anterior end of the inferior orbital fissure, a small groove may be noted for the passage of the zygomatic nerve and vessels. The groove often develops into a canal that divides within bone to conduct the zygomaticofacial vessels and nerves onto the face and the zygomaticotemporal vessels and nerves into the temporal fossa. The zygomaticofacial and zygomaticotemporal complexes may pass through separate foramina.

The floor. The inferior orbital fissure (IOF) separates the greater sphenoid wing portion of the lateral wall from the floor. The fissure communicates with the pterygopalatine fossa as well as the infratemporal fossa. Through this fissure pass (1) the maxillary division of the trigeminal nerve, V2, and its branches; (2) the infraorbital artery; (3) branches of the sphenopalatine ganglion; and (4) branches of the inferior ophthalmic vein to the pterygoid plexus.

The thin orbital floor is composed of the orbital plate of the maxilla, the zygomatic bone anterolaterally, and the orbital process of the palatine bone posteriorly. A shallow rough area at the anteromedial angle (OBL) marks the origin of the inferior oblique muscle. The infraorbital groove runs forward from the inferior orbital fissure. Anteriorly, the groove becomes a canal within the maxilla, finally forming the infraorbital foramen on the face of the maxilla. The groove and canal transmit the infraorbital nerve and artery. From the lower aspect of this nerve, middle superior alveolar nerves (occasionally) emanate to supply the bicuspid teeth. More anteriorly and 5 to 20 mm prior to the infraorbital nerve exit from its foramen, the anterior superior alveolar nerves descend medially along the inner face of the maxilla or within a canal to supply sensation to the anterior three teeth and gingiva.

The medial wall. The medial wall is quadrangular in shape and is composed of four bones: (1) the ethmoid bone centrally; (2) the frontal bone superoanteriorly; (3) the lacrimal bone inferoanteriorly; and (4) the sphenoid bone posteriorly. The inferior orbital margin continues upward into the anterior lacrimal crest (ALC), part of the frontal process of the maxilla. The superomedial margin continues downward into the posterior lacrimal crest (PLC) part of the lacrimal bone. Between these rests the fossa for the lacrimal sac (LF). Usually, the fossa is approximately 14 mm in height.

The medial wall is quite thin, and the ethmoidal portion has been termed lamina papyracea. The anterior and posterior ethmoidal foramina (AE, PE) are noted at the frontoethmoidal suture and denote the level of the cribriform plate. The anterior ethmoidal foramen transmits the anterior ethmoidal artery and the anterior ethmoidal nerve branches of the nasociliary nerve. The posterior ethmoidal foramen provides a passage for the posterior ethmoidal artery and, occasionally, for a sphenoethmoidal nerve branch from the nasociliary nerve.

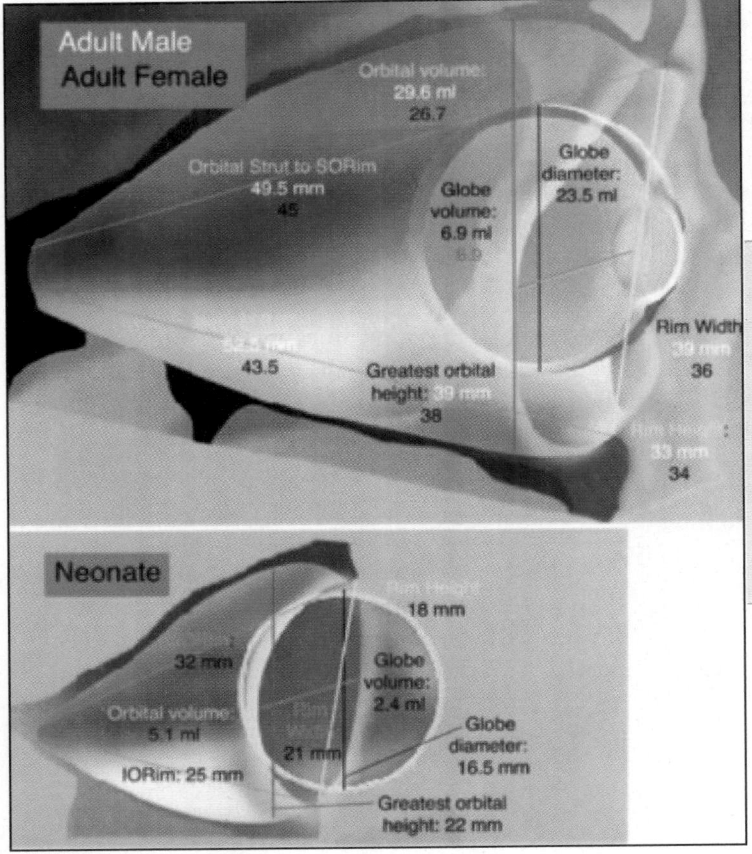

A

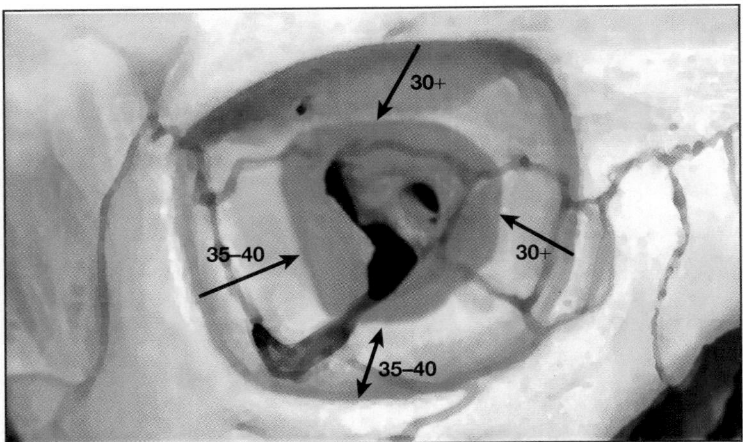

B

Figures 1.4 (A–B)

Volumes and distances: Males/females and babies

In theory, everything outside the annulus (Fig. 1.4A) and superior orbital fissure is safe. As the surgeon realizes the distance to the optic foramen is approximately 50 mm (men) and 45 mm (women) and gives at least 1 cm margin, the surgeon may dissect 35 to 40 mm back on the floor and roof region. Lateral dissection may even go a bit farther back.

Figure 1.5

The orbital width measures 39 to 45 mm. Note the infraorbital fissure (*dotted area*) where the infraorbital nerve travels. In this skull, the supraorbital nerve comes out a foramen (*right*) and a notch (*left*). Commentary: In this skull a ridge (*arrow*) is noted. It is quite common and should not be mistaken for a fracture on x-ray. Note also the deviation of the perpendicular ethmoid plate in the nose (*). The turbinate bone on the right is correspondingly larger also.

Note on anatomic variation: (L) infraorbital foramen is more lateral than usual.

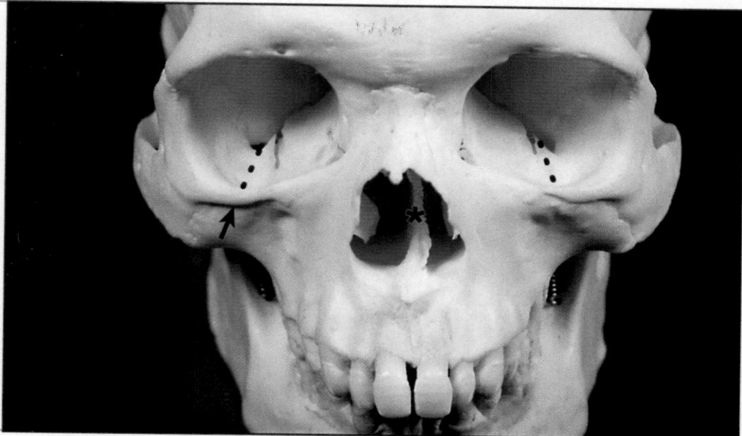

Figure 1.6 (A–D)

Topography 101

— Bony orbit (Fig. 1.6A)

— Medial to lateral 40 to 45 mm± (Fig. 1.6B)

(Figure continues on next page)

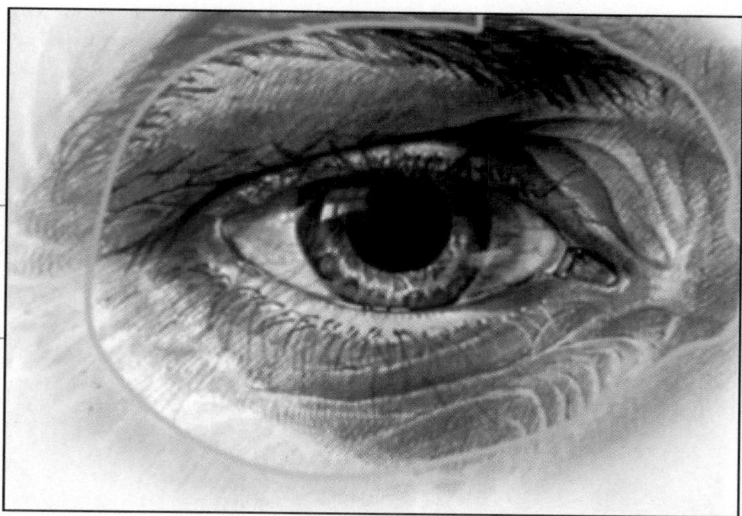

A

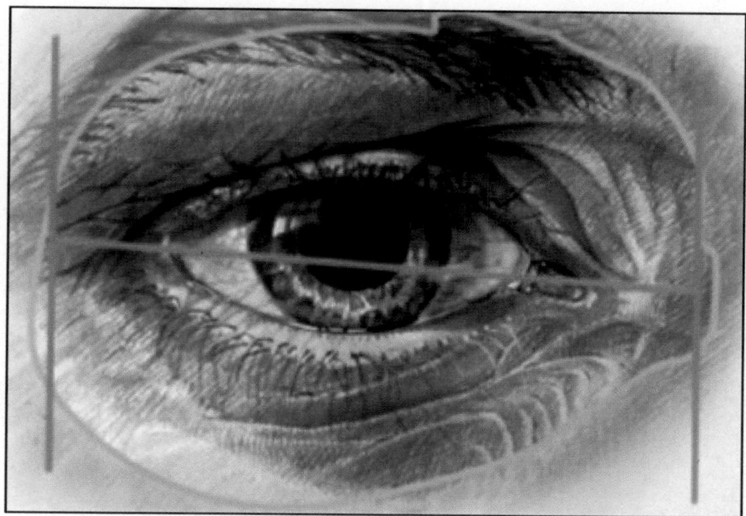

B

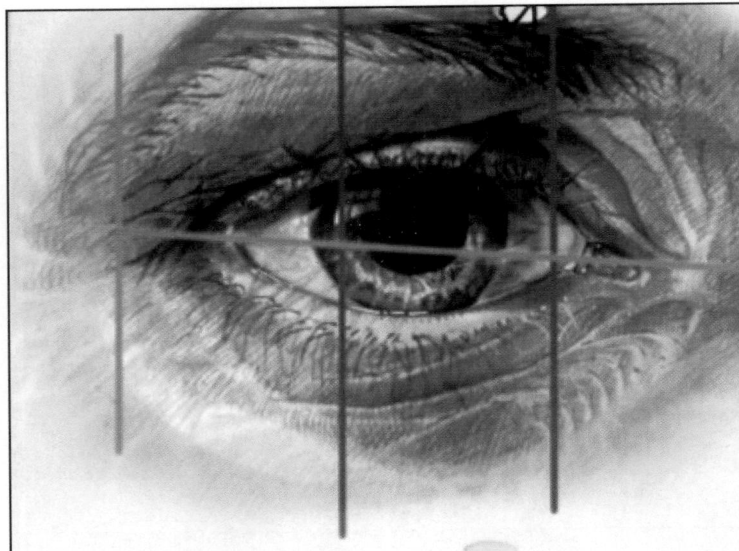

C

Figure. 1.6 (A–D) (continued)

— Bony orbit separated into thirds (~14.1 mm) by vertical purple. (Fig. 1.6C).

— Infraorbital foramen on line with medial limbus (*). Infraorbital foramen is approximately 5 to 7 mm below rim. Supraorbital nerve position varies 2.3 to 2.9 mm from midline and usually is a bit more medial than infraorbital (Fig. 1.6D).

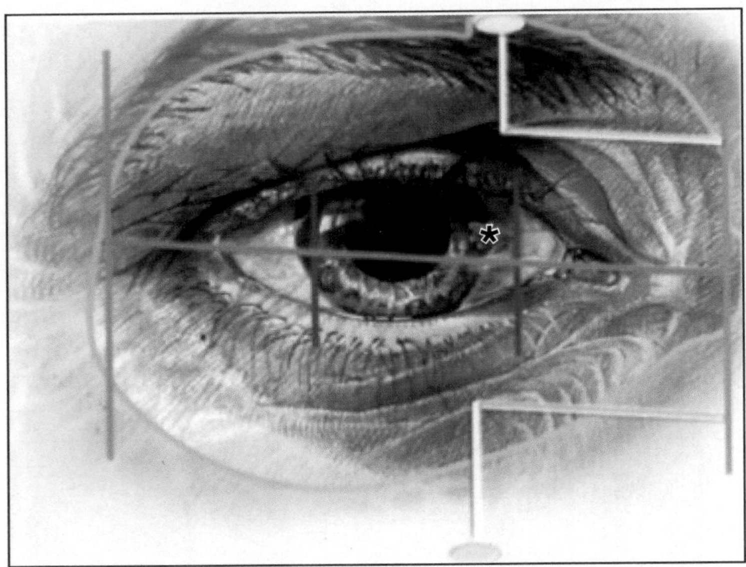

D

Figure 1.7

— The lacrimal bone (L) exists wholly within the orbital confines.

— A light is shining through the nose. There are holes in the medial and superior orbit. This still shows the extreme thinness of the medial wall. This thinness provides little protection from infections in the ethmoid air cells. The lesser thinness of the orbital floor which overlies the sinus is demonstrated. The optic foramen (circular) can be seen posteriorly and the fissure on the floor is noted (*).

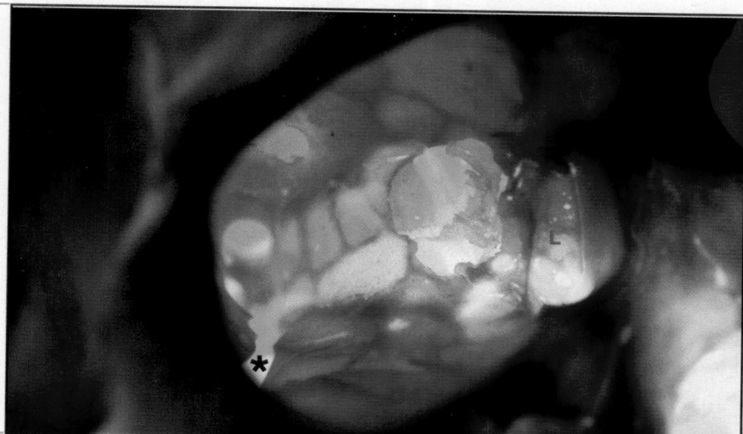

Figure 1.8

The angle between the lateral walls of both orbits is approximately 90 degrees. The angle between the lateral and medial walls of a single side is approximately 45 degrees. The two medial walls appear almost parallel. The orbital axis (OX) and visual axis (VX) do not coincide, but diverge at an angle of approximately 23 degrees. The orbital axis is the bisection line between the medial and lateral walls. The visual axis corresponds to the position of the eye in straight gaze.

On both sides of this skull, the medial and lateral branches exit separate holes. As noted and seen in the schematic, they travel on different planes. The medial supraorbital branch travels under the corrugator, pierces the frontalis, and then divides into multiple vertical supramuscular branches to supply the forehead and anterior scalp over the orbits. The deep branch (1–3) travels submuscular and subperiosteal, but always medial to the superior temporal line where the upper temporalis muscle arises.

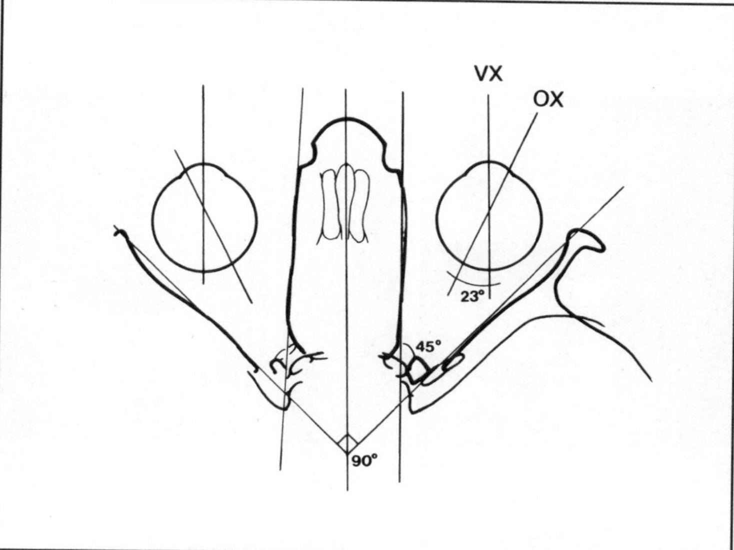

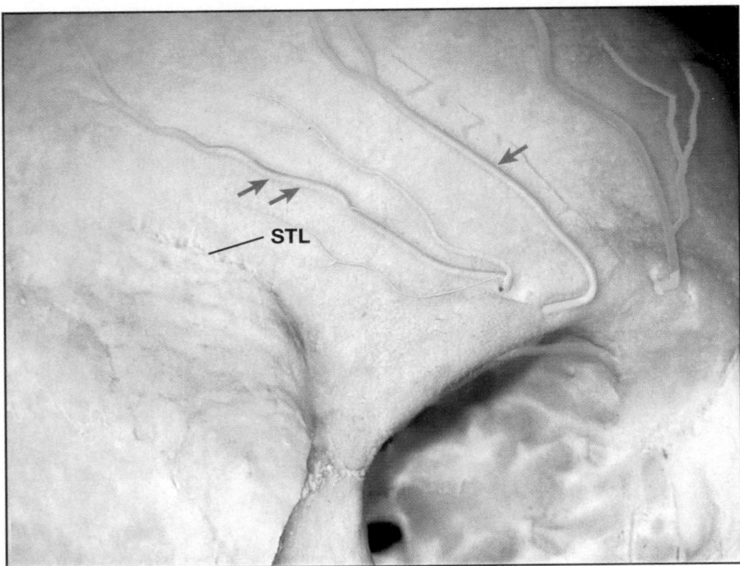

A

Figure 1.9A

The drawing shows the supraorbital nerve (medial or superficial branch arrow) which goes under the corrugator to pierce the frontalis and put branches that lie on top of frontalis muscle. The lateral branch (or deep branch [2 arrows]) may or may not exit from a separate hole, to become 1–3 branches traveling under the muscle to supply the superolateral forehead and scalp. Its foramen may vary in position, but they are always 0.5 to 1.0 cm or so medial to the superior temporal line (STL).

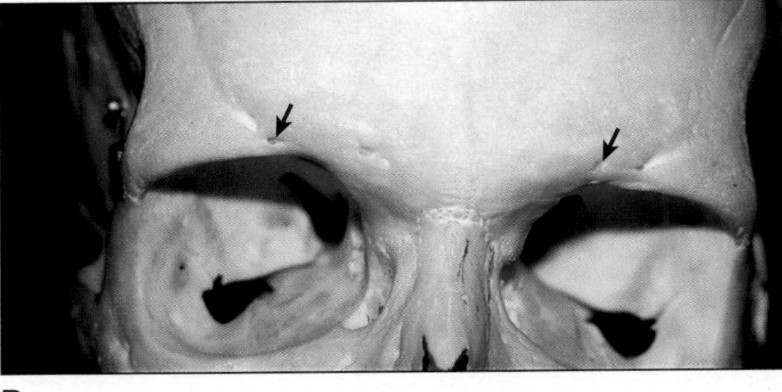

B

Figure 1.9B

The supraorbital nerve may exit via a notch in the upper rim or via a foramen or foramina. If both the lateral and medial branches exit together via a notch, the arcus marginalis or a fascial band will be under the nerve. When the nerve exits a foramen (or foramina), the medial and lateral branches may exit separately or together. The lateral branch may exit via one or more holes to travel obliquely upward below the muscle. There may be one to three branches which all travel medially toward the superior temporal line. Sometimes there are some subperiosteal branches, as well, and a groove may be noted as in this specimen. These lateral branches supply sensation to the lateral forehead into the scalp.

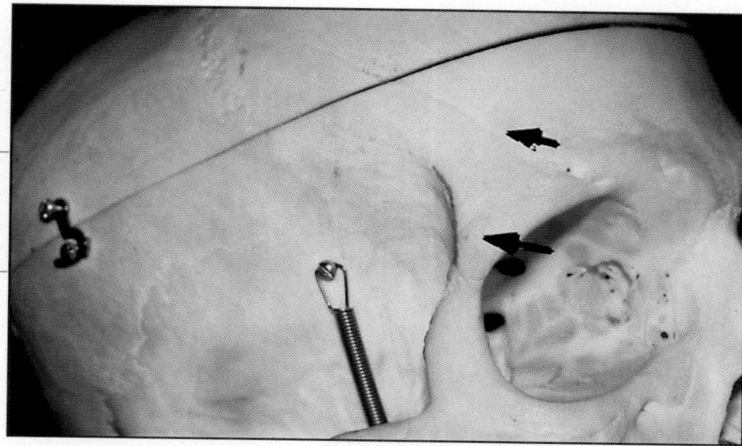

Figure 1.9C

The lower arrow shows the region where the lacrimal nerve comes from inside to around the superolateral rim to supply skin sensation there.

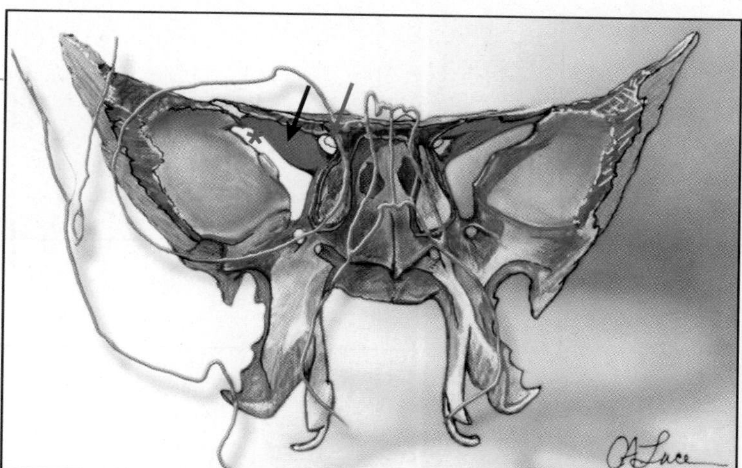

Figure 1.10

The keystone to the bony orbit is the sphenoid bone, shown here from its anterior aspect. All neurovascular structures to the orbit pass through this bone. The superior orbital fissure (*) is the gap between the lesser wing (*arrow*) and the greater wing (*light blue*) of the sphenoid bone. The optic canal (*red arrow*) is medial to the superior orbital fissure within the substance of the lesser wing.

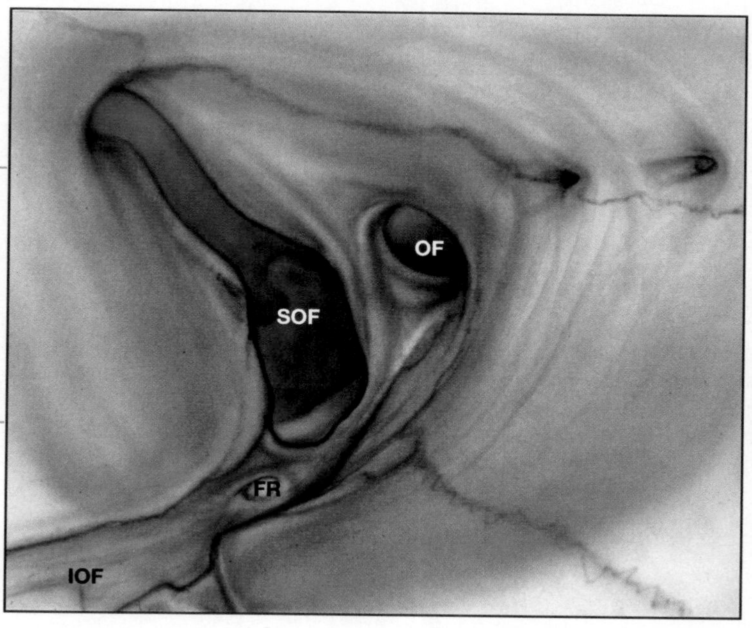

Figure 1.11

The superior orbital fissure widens medially where it lies below the level of the optic foramen (OF). Note the foramen rotundum (FR) just inferior to the confluence between the superior orbital fissure (SOF) and inferior orbital fissure (IOF). The total length of the superior orbital fissure is 22 mm.

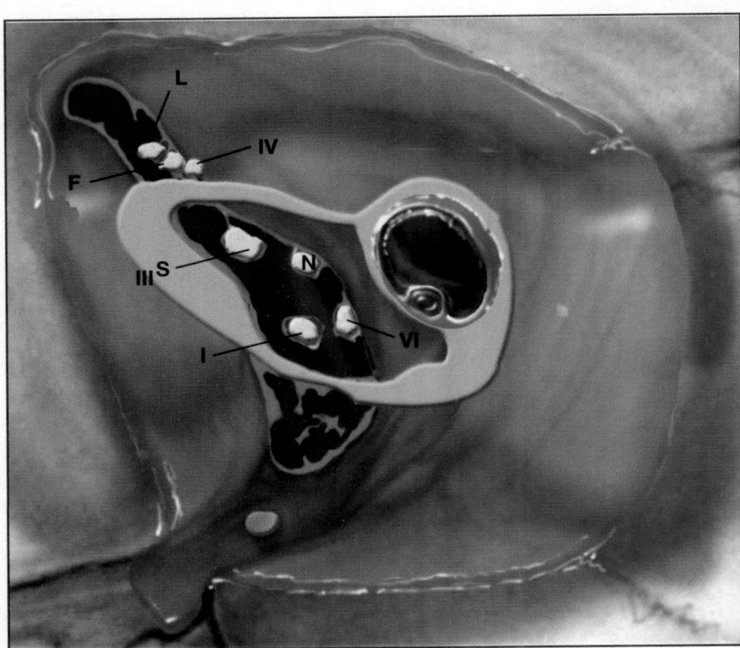

Figure 1.12A

The common tendinous ring, or annulus of Zinn, divides the superior orbital fissure. The extraocular muscles arise from this common ring. The portion of the annulus that is formed by the origin of the lateral rectus muscle divides the superior orbital fissure into two compartments. That area encircled by the annulus is termed the oculomotor foramen, which opens into the middle cranial fossa and transmits (1) cranial nerve III (upper [s] and lower divisions [I]); (2) cranial nerve VI; (3) the nasociliary branch of cranial nerve V; (4) ophthalmic veins; (5) the orbital branch of the middle meningeal artery (occasionally); and (6) sympathetic nerve fibers. Above the annulus, note the trochlear nerve (IV) and the frontal (F) and lacrimal (L) branches of cranial nerve V. It is important to realize that the frontal and lacrimal branches of the ophthalmic division of cranial nerve V and the trochlear nerve enter the orbit outside the muscle cone.

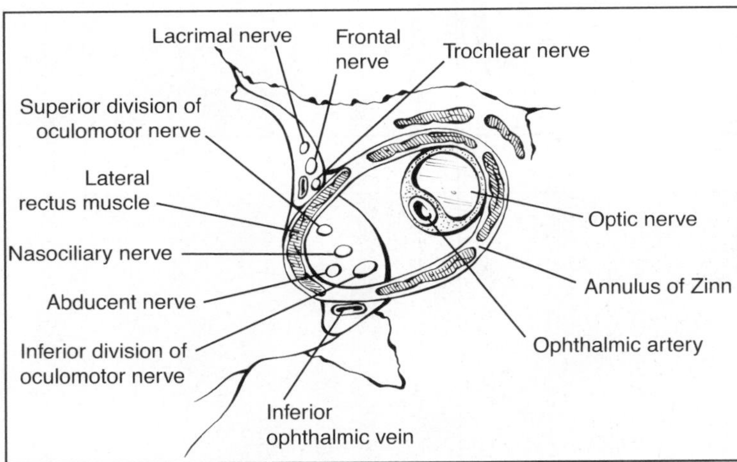

Figure 1.12B

Posterior orbit: The annulus of Zinn.

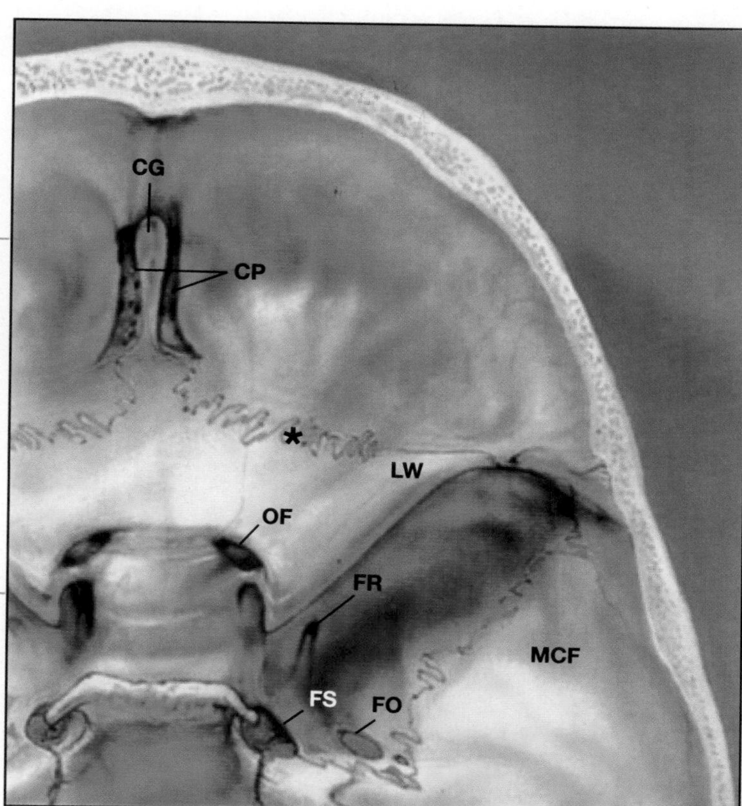

Figure 1.13A

The skullcap is removed to expose the roof of the right orbit. For orientation, note the crista galli (CG), straddled by paired cribriform plates (CP). The optic foramen (OF) may be seen within the lesser wing of the sphenoid bone (LW). The frontosphenoidal sutures (*) separate frontal bone from the more posterior sphenoid bone. The foramen rotundum (FR), foramen spinosum (FS), and foramen ovale (FO) are noted within the middle cranial fossa (MCF).

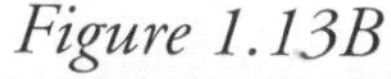

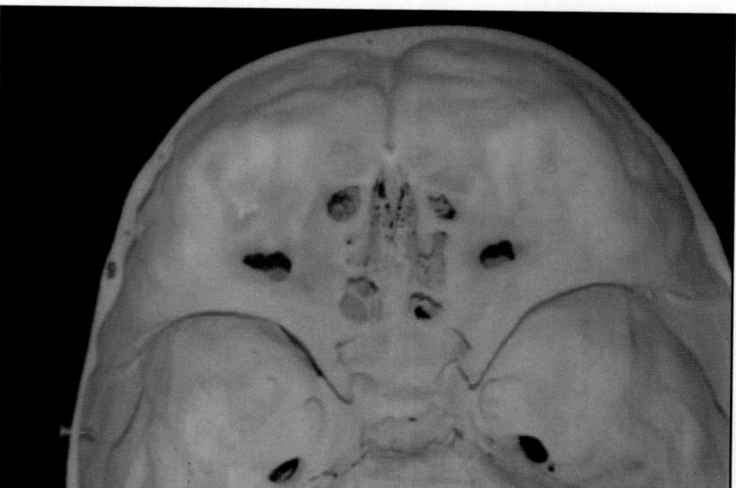

Figure 1.13B

A typical skull with thin orbital roof on both sides.

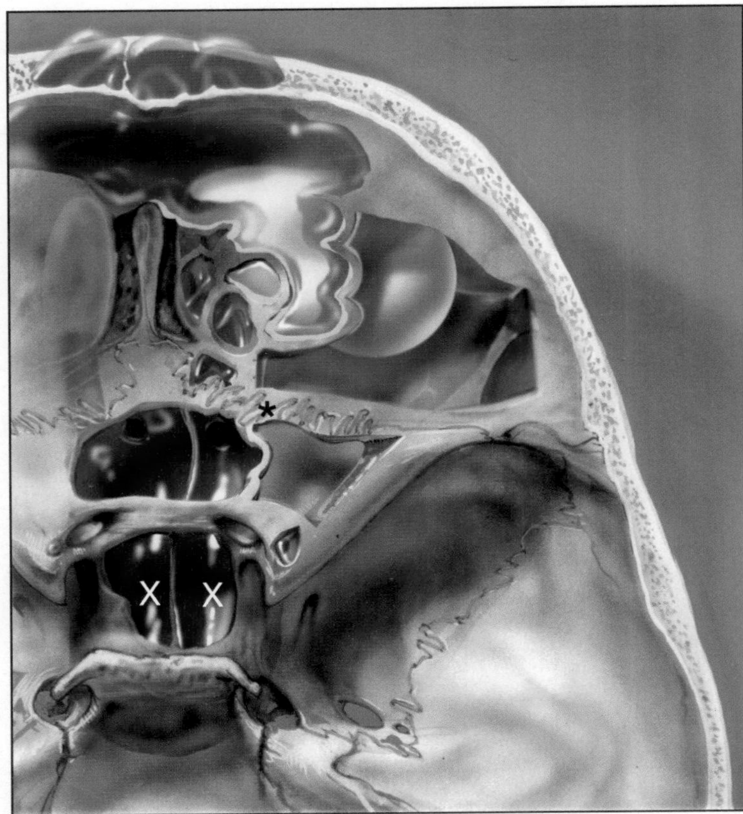

Figure 1.14

The roof of the orbit is removed except for the frontosphenoid suture (*). The sinuses are marked as follows: frontal sinus (*green*); anterior ethmoidal air cells; posterior ethmoidal air cells (*purple*); and sphenoid sinus (X).

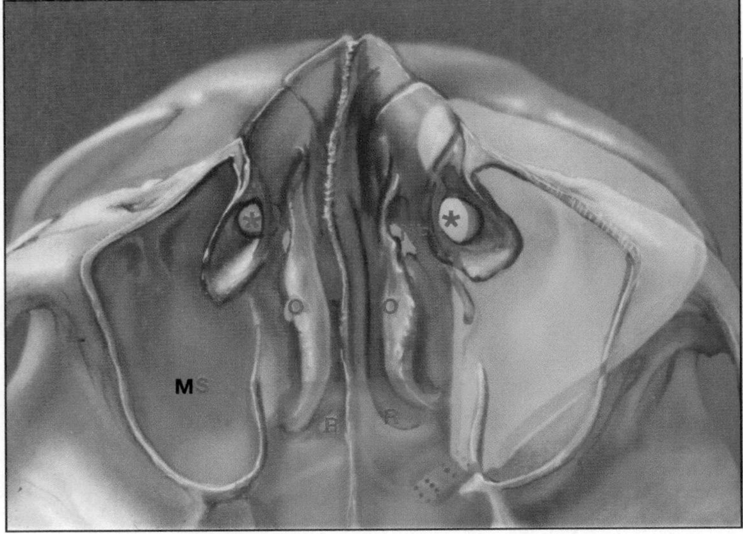

Figure 1.15

The maxillary sinuses (MS) are exposed after transverse section below the orbits. The transected nasolacrimal canals (*), which later empty into the inferior meati, are noted medially on each side. The nasofrontal ducts (NF) empty into the anterior portion of the middle meati most commonly. The ethmoidal ostia (O) usually enter the nose in the middle meatus at its midportion. The sphenoid sinuses empty into the nose at the sphenoethmoid recesses (R). The relative position of the cribriform plate is noted (*magenta*).

Figure 1.16

Note: Vol. I: *Surgical Anatomy of the Orbit* has named even the smaller branches. Here, though, I am focusing on the surrounding region and something new, as noted in the second drawing and the artery comment sheet.

1. Internal maxillary
2. Internal carotid
3. Frontal branch of superficial temporal
4. Middle meningeal
5. Transverse facial
6. Facial artery
7. Angular artery
8. Infraorbital artery
9. Zygomatic artery
10. Zygomaticotemporal
11. Zygomaticofacial

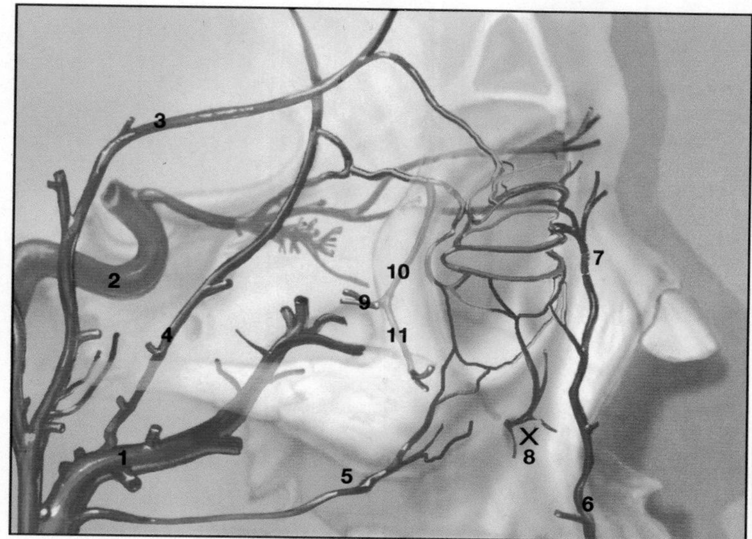

Figure 1.17

In the upper lid, there exists a marginal arcade (M) along the eyelid border and a peripheral arcade (P) above the tarsus but below the levator aponeurosis. More recently two other arcades, one above and one below the orbicularis, have been noted up near the rim. No such arcades have been found inferiorly. The superficial (S) and deep (D) arcades are noted.

In the upper lid laterally a lacrimal artery branch and medially a medial palpebral artery contribute to the upper lid's lower arcades. They are not drawn to simplify things. Also not drawn is the medial inferior palpebral artery of lower lid.

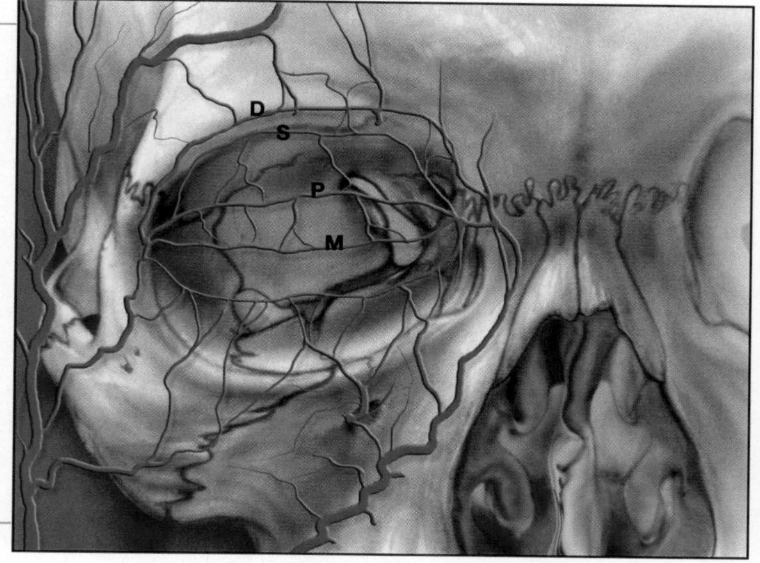

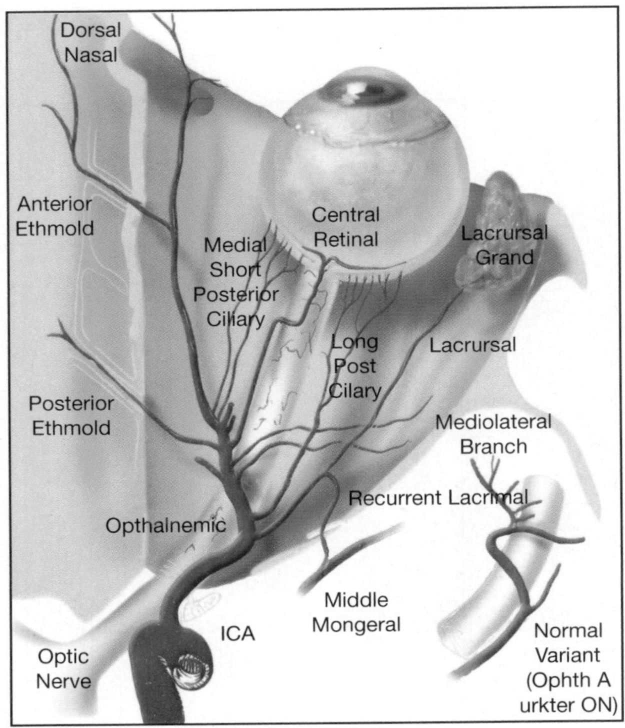

Figure 1.18 Upper lid arteries and vessels along the superior orbitol rim

Upper lid arteries and vessels along the superior orbital rim

When dissecting from above via endoscope, the supraorbital nerve area may yield *venous* bleeding, profuse at times. The supratrochlear region, though, has defined arteries that supply the paramedian forehead flap, usually "Dopplered" 1.5 to 2.3 cm from the midline. Arterial bleeding rarely occurs during bicoronal or endoscopic work, however. Excellent work from Japan had defined this area better from an arterial vascular standpoint. (See Figure 1.17.)

There are four upper-lid arterial arcades. You already know about the following two:

1. The **marginal arcade** courses along the pretarsal, submuscular eyelid, just above the lid margin. This arcade anastomoses via branches to the other three.
2. The **peripheral arcade** courses in Müllers muscle along the upper border of the tarsal plate.

The newer arcades consist of the superficial orbital arcade (SOA) and the deep orbital arcade (DOA).

As the frontal branch of the superficial temporal, the transverse facial, and zygomatico-orbital arteries course toward the lateral upper eyelid, these latter two arcades are formed which anastomose medially with the supratrochlear, and receive vertical contributions from the marginal and peripheral arcades.

When the branches of the marginal arcade course upward *on the surface* of the orbicularis oculi, they join the SOA.

The branches that course vertically posterior to the orbicularis muscle, branch with the DOA beneath the muscle.

The orbicularis itself does not have an intramuscular vessel; rather, it gets branches from the vertical plexuses going upward from the arcade and downward from the higher ones.

The SOA (above) and the DOA (below), which course lateral to medial with muscle in between, exist near the orbital rim, continuing to join the supratrochlear vessels.

Figure 1.19 Sensory nerves

1. Trigeminal ganglion
2. V1 division of trigeminal nerve
3. V2 division of trigeminal nerve
4. Frontal nerve
5. Supraorbital nerve
6. Supratrochlear nerve
7. Infratrochlear nerve
8. Anterior ethmoidal nerve (posterior ethmoidal often lacking)
9. Dorsal nerve
10. Infraorbital nerve
11. Zygomaticofacial nerve(s)
12. Zygomaticotemporal nerve
13. Lacrimal nerve
14. Zygomatic nerve

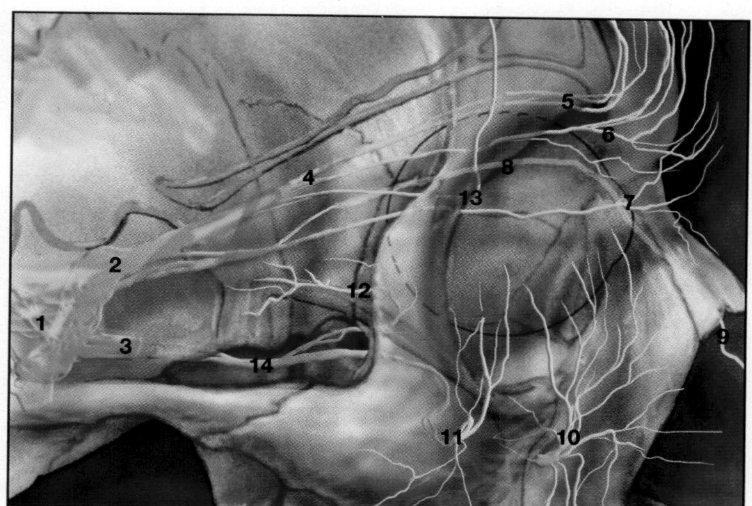

Figure 1.20 Sensory branches within the orbit

1. Short ciliary nerve
2. Long ciliary nerve
3. Nerve to inferior oblique (off inferior division of oculomotor)
4. Ciliary ganglion
5. Nasociliary nerve

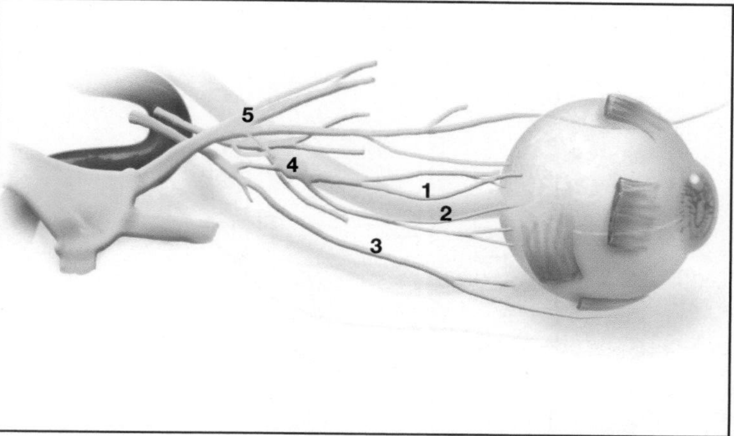

CHAPTER 2

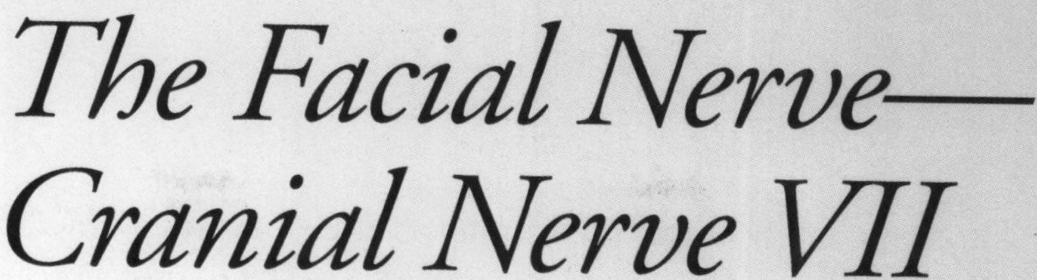

The Facial Nerve—Cranial Nerve VII

Many of the advances in surgical and frontal techniques have forced the surgeon to understand the course of the temporal and zygomatic branches exactly. The following pictures present crucial data that involve the correlation of many studies. The numbers must be absorbed, yet the surgeon must understand that absolutes never exist in anatomy. Clinical injection studies depict the real-life effects of nerve loss, and a case will validate that study.

I have taken the liberty of making certain safety decisions. For example, if a study shows the facial nerve between 3.5 and 4.5 cm from a point, I always chose the *closest* number, so the surgeon would have some margin of protection.

Data to read and reread after reviewing the upcoming pictures:

1. Two to five facial nerve branches cross the zygomatic arch. These are the frontal or temporal branches of cranial nerve VII.
2. These nerves cross the arch between 0.8 and 3.5 cm anterior to the external acoustic canal (EAC). At 2.5 cm from the EAC, branches can always be found just above the periosteum on the arch.
3. The most anterior temporal branch provides motor to the upper lid orbicularis oculi, entering the orbicularis oculi *2.1 to 3.5 cm* above the bony lateral canthus (average: 2.8 cm).
4. A safe zone can be designated starting at the zygomatic arch anteriorly. The first 2 cm posterior to the lower lateral orbit rim (actually, the lateral border of the orbital portion of the zygoma) is safe at the arch level.
5. At the level of the bony lateral canthus over the temporalis fascia, the most anterior branch is at least *3.5 cm* away (3.9 ± 0.4 cm).

6 The nerve rarely enters the frontalis muscle beyond 4 cm above the bony lateral canthus, or usually 2 cm above the lateral brow. The brow is a less reliable anatomic point.

7 The frontal branch of the superficial temporal artery can often be noted in the lateral forehead and can be used to mark the highest possible nerve entrance into the frontalis muscle.

8 The safe zone at 3.5 cm can be marked "digitally" along the rim during sub SMAS surgery (Fig. 2.14) to allow for safe transection of ligaments that go to the skin under the superficial musculo-aponeurotic system (SMAS) layer (see Fig. 2.15).

9 The bare zygomatic arch or deep temporal fascia can be safely exposed anteriorly in the 2-cm zone behind the rim. Posterior to that, a cut in the fascia where it splits to envelop the arch is required to get to the back of the arch without any nerve injury. A similar posterior approach behind the front leaf of split fascia can be used to reach the posterior arch, and subperiosteal elevation can be performed over the arch.

10 The zygomatic branch supplies the lower lid muscle and the zygomaticus muscles and lip levators anterior to that. The zygomatic branch also curves around the lower lid to supply the medial upper lid depressors. The depressor supercilii and the medial orbicularis in the upper lid on the same side are supplied by the zygomatic branches as they curve around the canthal region.

11 The orbicularis oculi muscle (upper) is usually supplied by the most anterior temporal branch to cross the zygomatic arch. Motor shoots to the lower orbicularis oculi from the zygomatic branch often separate proximally either within or just outside the parotid to cross the arch into the deep fat before going to supply the muscle. This branch starts *prior* to the zygomaticocutaneous ligaments. The main zygomatic branch, however, just below the zygomaticocutaneous ligaments provides key nerves to the orbicularis oculi just before passing to the deep side of the zygomaticus major, which it supplies. This branch continues on to the surface of the zygomaticus minor (supplying it) and becomes more vertical.

Thus, the lower orbicularis muscle has transverse nerve fibers to it from the zygomatic branch which may explain why leaving this pretarsal muscle (innervated) may be helpful during blepharoplasty. Also, the preseptal and orbital fibers have vertical fibers supplying it from the zygomatic branch of cranial nerve VII.

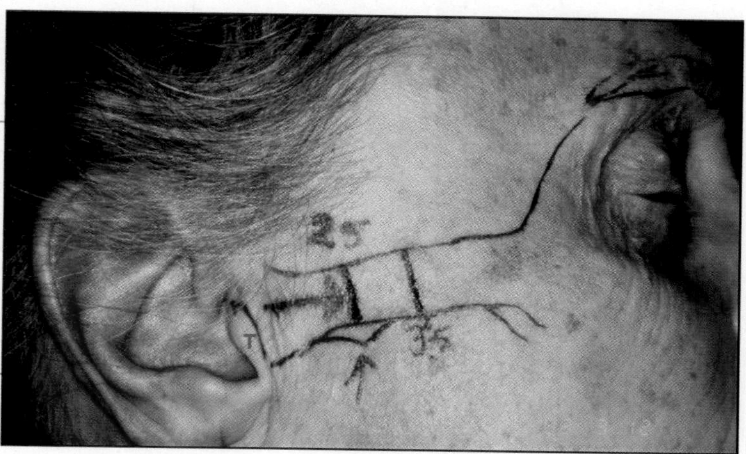

Figure 2.1

The purple line along the anterior tragus (T) is the front of the external acoustic canal (EAC). Most of the cranial nerve VII branches can be found about 2.5 cm in front of the EAC (range: 0.8 cm to 3.5 cm). The lower arrow shows the articular eminence to be at about 2.5 cm from the anterior border of the canal.

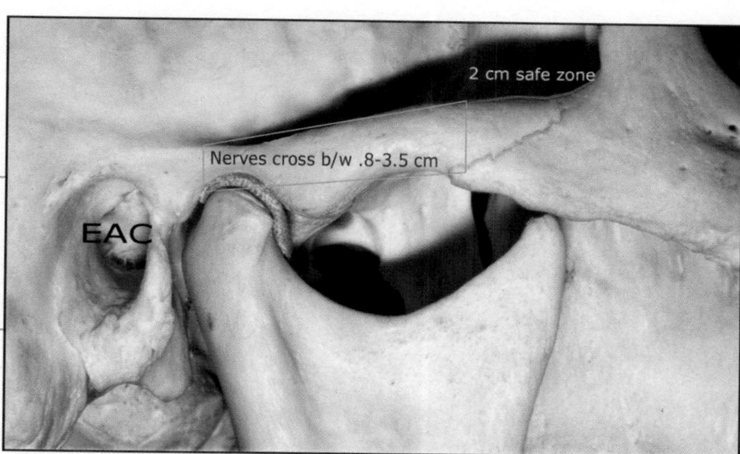

Figure 2.2

Along the upper arch anteriorly, for the 2 cm posterior to the lateral orbital rim, there are no key nerves, so this area and the fascia above are safe for sutures for that 2-cm distance.

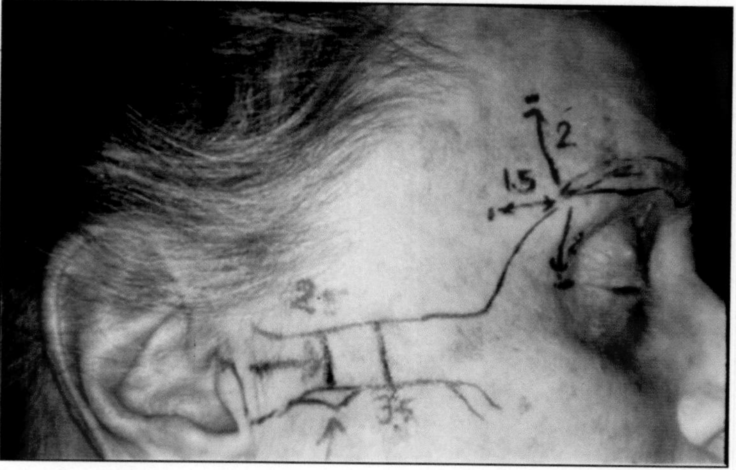

Figure 2.3

The eyebrow is a soft reference point. Therefore, saying the nerve is usually 1.5 cm lateral to it also becomes soft information.

Note the horizontal line above the 2 on the forehead. Here, the anterior branch of the superficial temporal artery can often be palpated in vivo. The nerves are practically below the artery, usually in the first 2 cm above the lateral brow. Rarely are the nerves beyond 4 cm from the bony lateral canthus (horizontal line lateral to canthus).

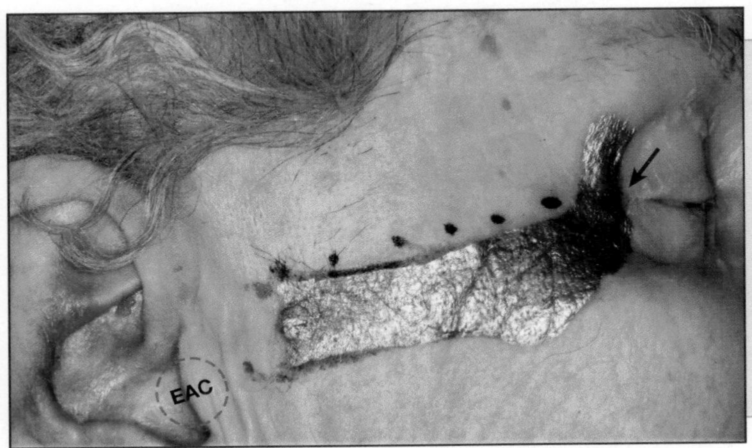

Figure 2.4

1. The bone is marked with silver.
2. Posterior red dot is 8 mm from the EAM (external acoustic meatus) or EAC.
3. Anterior red dot (canal) (*arrow*) appears at the bony lateral canthus.
4. Black dots connect the red dots and follow the upper arch closely. Note that the horizontal width of the lateral orbital rim prior to its turn back to become arch is about 1.3 cm to 1.5 cm.

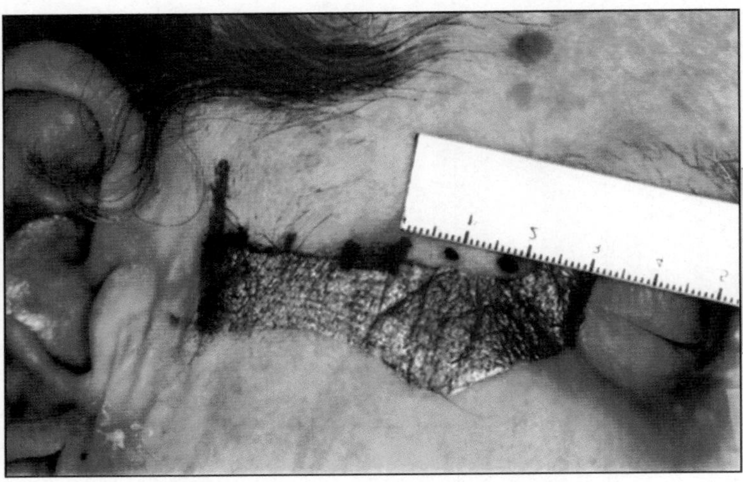

Figure 2.5

The first 2 cm behind the lateral orbital rim is a *safe area*. The long vertical blue line is at 0.8 cm. The most anterior vertical blue line is at 3.5 cm. Nerves are always between the front and back blue lines.

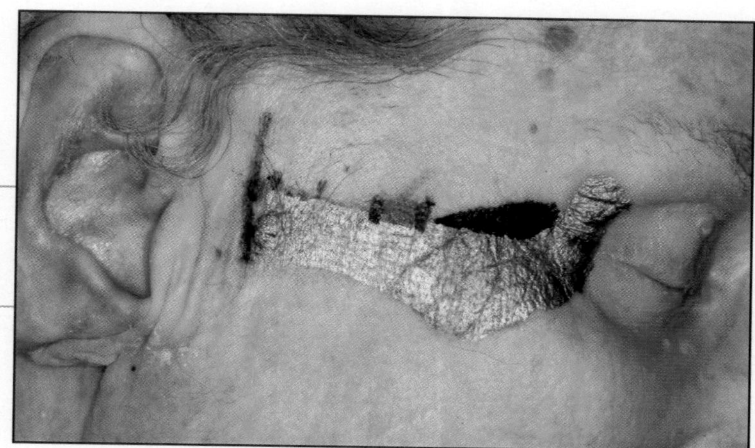

Figure 2.6

The black fill indicates the start of marking a *safe zone* 2 cm behind the lateral orbital rim (LOR).

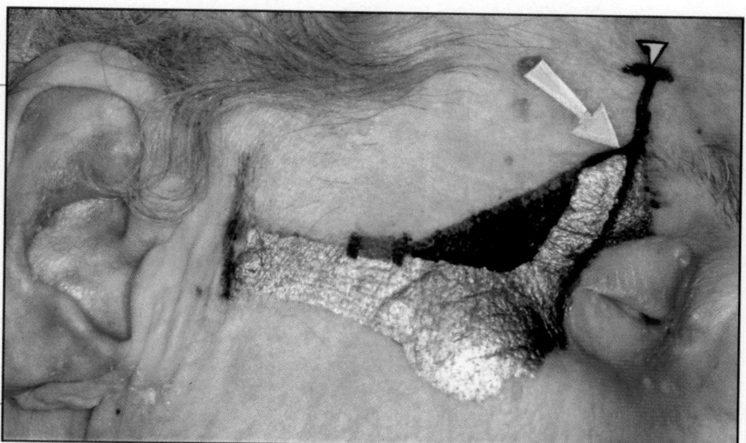

Figure 2.7

The highest point where the nerve enters the frontalis (*yellow/black dart*) is at least 4 cm above the bony lateral canthus (*red dot*) (range 2.85 ± 0.7 cm). The height of the yellow arrow at 2.85 cm above the bony canthus is the level where the most anterior branch enters the orbicularis oculi lateral border. Note, however, that the orbicularis border is *more than* 1 cm lateral to this point, as you will see.

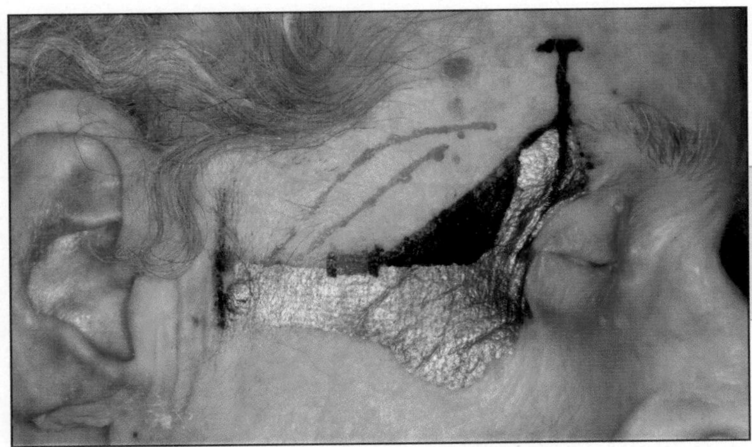

Figure 2.8A

The red lines show that the nerve's pathways may be relatively straight or curved as shown. The red lines stop at the point where the anterior branch would enter the upper orbicularis oculi.

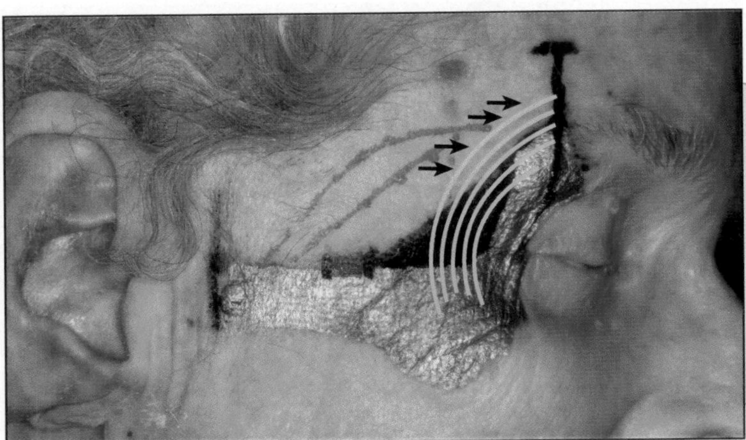

B

Figure 2.8B

The longer arrow in Figure 2.7 shows the average height at which the most anterior branch of the frontal group enters the orbicularis. In fact, its from 2.1 to 3.5 cm from the bony canthus. If the orbucularis oculi muscle is then ghosted in (*orange brown*), the arrows then depict the possible entrance of the anterior branch into the upper lid orbicularis. See Figures 2.10B, 2.12, and 2.13 for actual dissections of this.

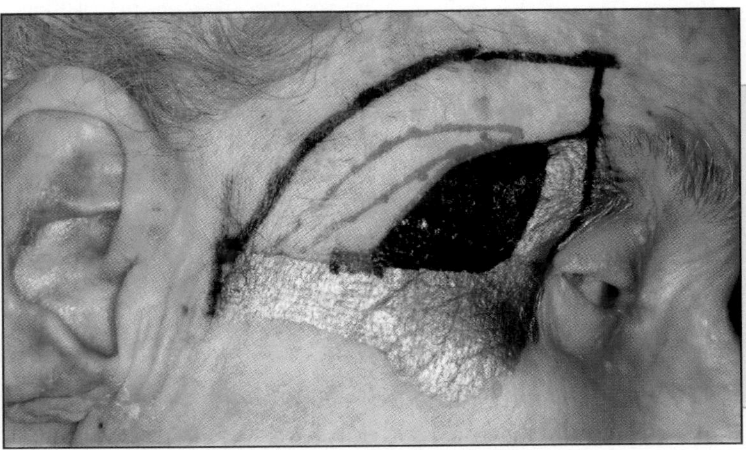

Figure 2.9

Silver dots indicate the most anterior nerve at the level of the canthus. The closest the most anterior branch ever is to the bony canthus at the canthal level is 4.3 cm ± .0.8 cm. *Dots*: 3.5 cm from the bony lateral canthus. *Black*: safe zone completed. *Blue line, curved*: posterior-most pathway for nerves. The shape of the safe zone and the shape of the nerve zones are now well demarcated.

Figure 2.10A

Skin removed: The frontal branch of the superficial temporal artery may be straight or tortuous, as noted, but the final point over the brow is always about 2.0 to 2.4 cm above it, and the frontal branches are almost always below the artery. Thus, we have seen that the nerves may take a straight or somewhat curved course, and likewise the artery may be straight or tortuous.

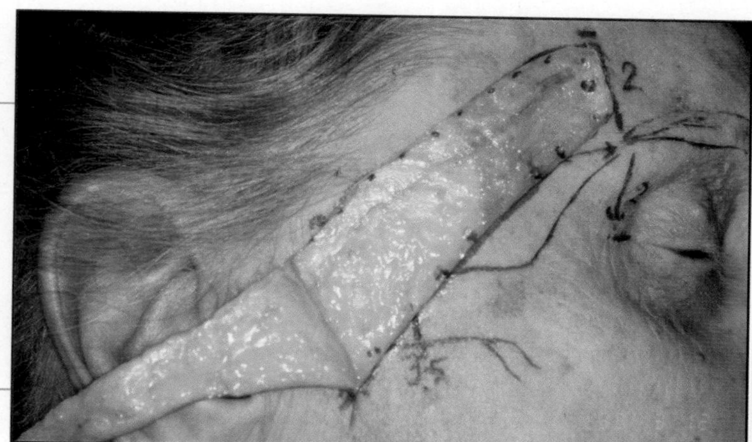

A

Figure 2.10B

The frontal branch of the artery is tortuous here. Note the position of the lateral part of orbital portion of the orbicularis oculi muscle. The arrows depict the zone where the most anterior branch of the nerve might enter from 2.1 to 3.5 (average 2.8 cm) above the bony lateral canthus (*red dot*).

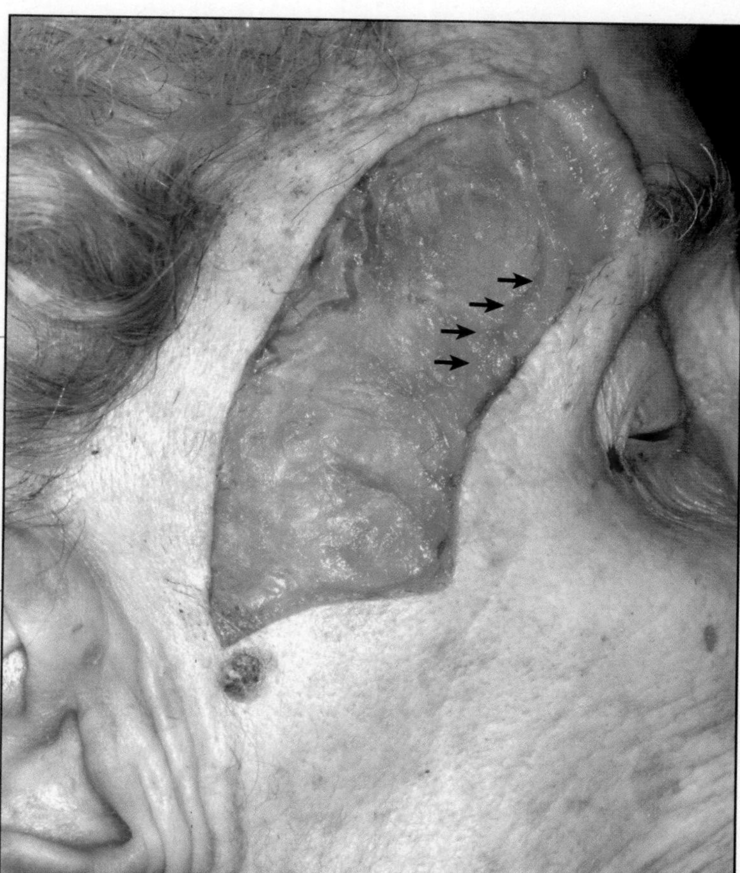

B

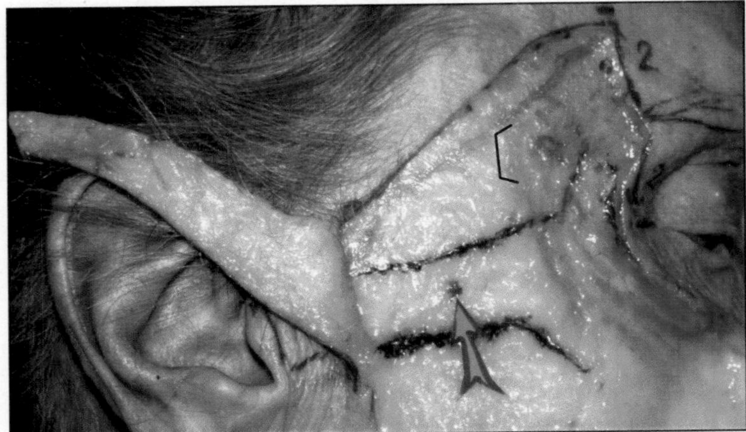

Figure 2.11

Arrow to dot is placed exactly 3.5 cm anterior to the EAM. Note the orbicularis ring around the lateral orbit. The surgeon might guess exactly where the most anterior branch would enter the orbicularis (⌐).

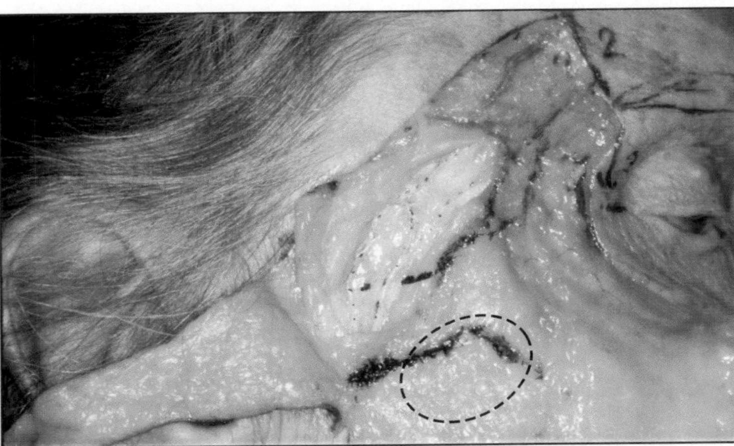

Figure 2.12

Branches of seventh nerve cross the arch. The anterior branch enters the orbicularis oculi to supply closing motor to the upper lid at just over 2 cm above the canthus in this case. Injury to this most anterior branch might thus affect the orbicularis (which has multiple other branches), but not the frontalis. A dotted zone is marked where the zygomaticocutaneous ligaments are usually found, anterior to the 3.5 cm mark (•).

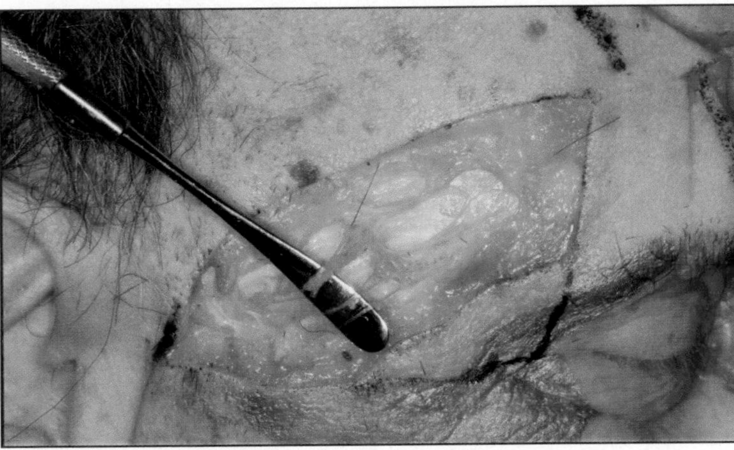

Figure 2.13

Two to five branches usually cross the arch in the noted zone. As the most anterior branch goes to the orbicularis, the surgeon usually has a few millimeters leeway prior to the frontal branches, which innervate the frontalis, corrugator, and procerus.

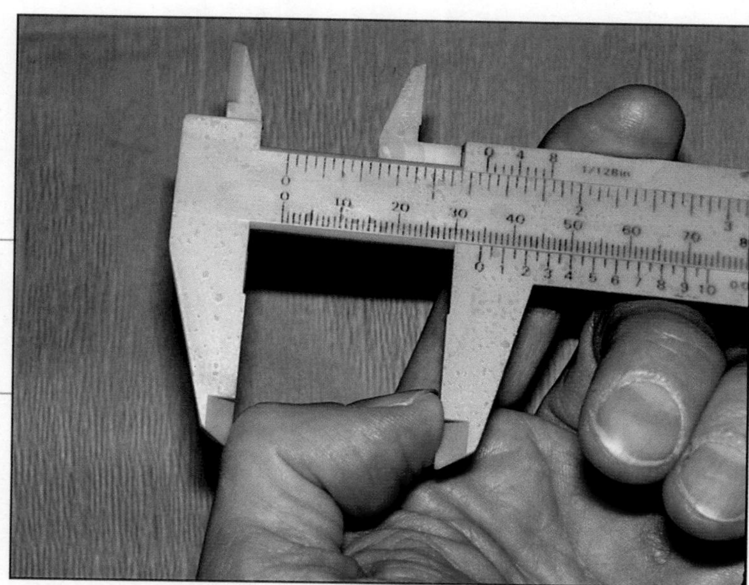

Figure 2.14

Digital ruler: Parts of your hand can be used for surgical purposes, e.g., for my hand, the distance noted is 3.5 cm from tip to interphalangeal thumb joint.

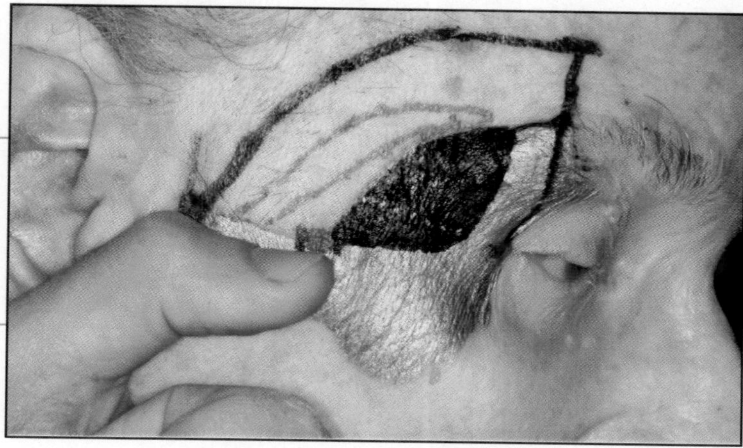

Figure 2.15

This can be used intraoperatively while dissecting under the SMAS. Any vertical ligament anterior to the thumb laid along the arch can be cut with impunity. This will be seen in other dissections.

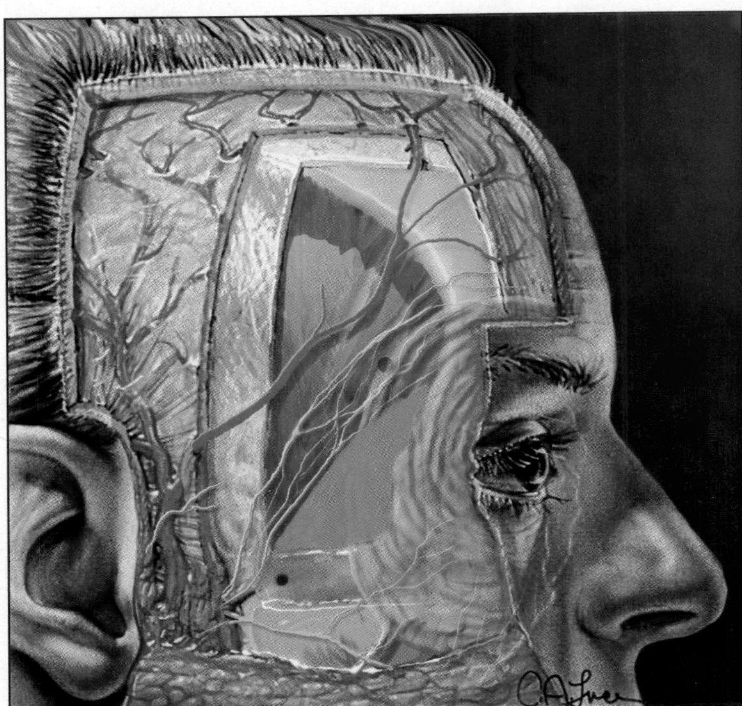

Figure 2.16

1. Just in front of the ear, the small auriculotemporal branch of V2 is noted over the superficial temporal artery or vein. This supplies sensation to the scalp above and around the sideburn.
2. The anterior branch of the superficial temporal artery is noted piercing the frontalis about 2.5 cm above the orbital rim. The facial nerves that enter the frontalis are always below the artery.
3. Two to five branches (temporal) cross the zygoma between 0.8 and 3.5 cm (*lower blue dot*) from the EAM (external acoustic meatus). (The EAM is not shown.)
4. The upper blue dot is the sentinel vein, which can be seen on endoscopy or via bicoronal incisions. Usually the frontal branches reside around this area; transection of this vein may yield more swelling postoperatively, but this is ultimately only an anatomic finding.
5. The most anterior facial nerve branch usually goes to the upper orbicularis muscle, which it enters laterally about 2.0 to 3.5 cm above the bony canthus.
6. As the most anterior branch is found usually at least 3.8 cm laterally to the bony canthus, a safe zone (*green*) can be noted.
7. The more anterior branches tend to be adherent to periosteum, whereas the posterior ones may have a little space between them and the periosteum (not shown).
8. The whitish deep temporal fascia always splits a couple of centimeters above the zygomatic arch that it envelopes (*not shown*), which may be found between the split leaves of fascia.

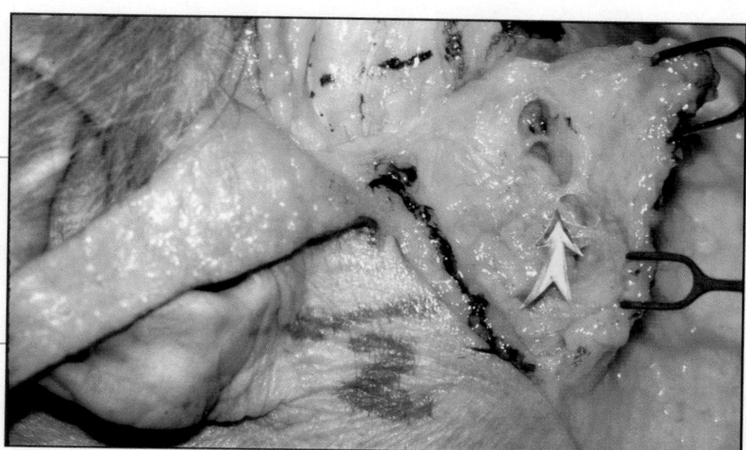

Figure 2.17

The SMAS is elevated with hooks. Ligaments to it which continue to skin can be seen (*arrow*). The nerves (*dotted*) are present posteriorly. Some parotid gland can be seen under the arrow in this dissection.

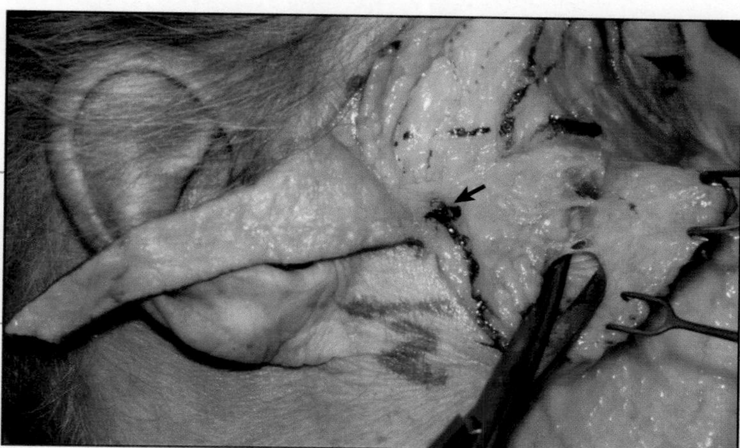

Figure 2.18

Vertical spreading always leaves any nerves on the down side, whether here or sub-SMAS inferiorly in the cheek. The seventh nerve is dotted mark on arch at 3.5 cm from the EAC (*arrow*).

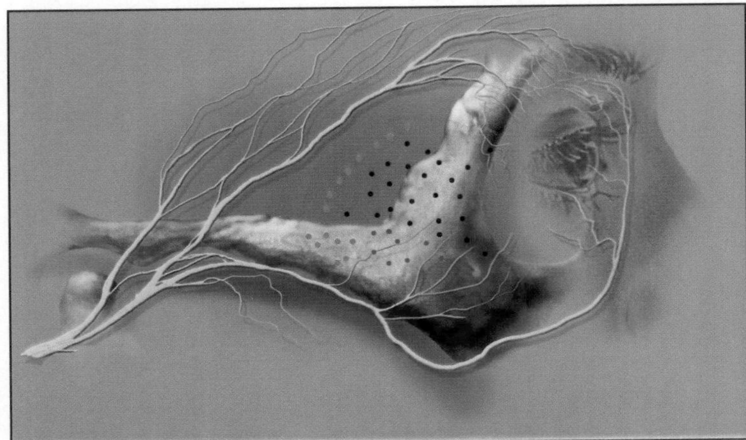

Figure 2.19

The light green opaque area denotes the deep temporal fascia (DTF) and the periosteum where sutures may be used to suspend soft tissue.

The black dots denote an area where orbicularis muscle can be sutured to support the lower lid. The lower black dots should be used when wide or extensive undermining (e.g., sutures to suborbucularis oculi fat) has been performed for additional lower lid support. Two or three absorbable sutures will make ectropion almost impossible with judicious support. The upper black dots are often used for drill holes or access to the DTF through the rim for canthopexy.

The blue dots—and posterior to them for 2 cm—is where the SMAS can be safely sutured to periosteum or fascia with or without bony anchors. In the red dot area, the surgeon approaches nerves, but is still safe.

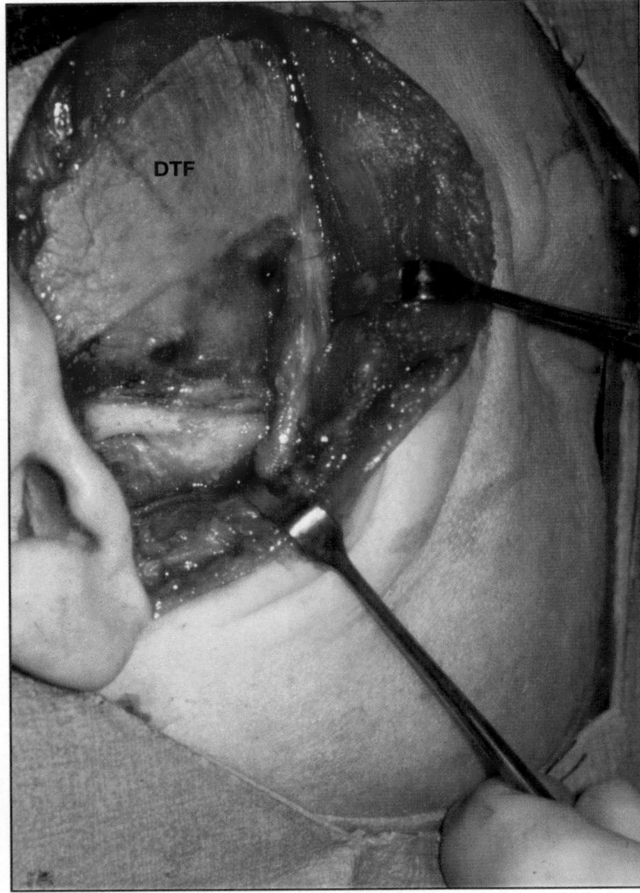

Figure 2.20

To approach the arch from behind, a slanted cut in the deep temporal fascia allows the surgeon to get to the upper posterior arch after cutting along the anterior edge. With subperiosteal dissection, the nerves can be safely pushed off the arch. Of course the cut into periosteum is behind the anterior leave of deep temporal fascia after it splits. (Courtesy Michael F. Zide, DMD)

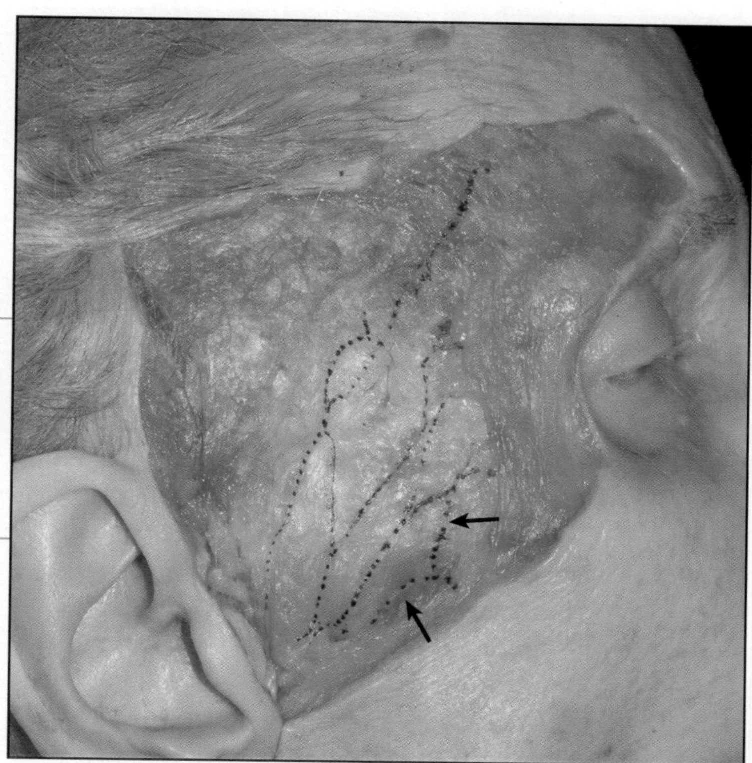

Figure 2.21

Nerve branches (*dotted*). Nerves cross the arch and follow the "prescribed path." Anteriorly, the zygomatic branch (*arrow*) curves below the arch, but first gives a small branch to the orbicularis oculi (*upper arrow*). Connections can be seen between the temporal and zygomatic branches.

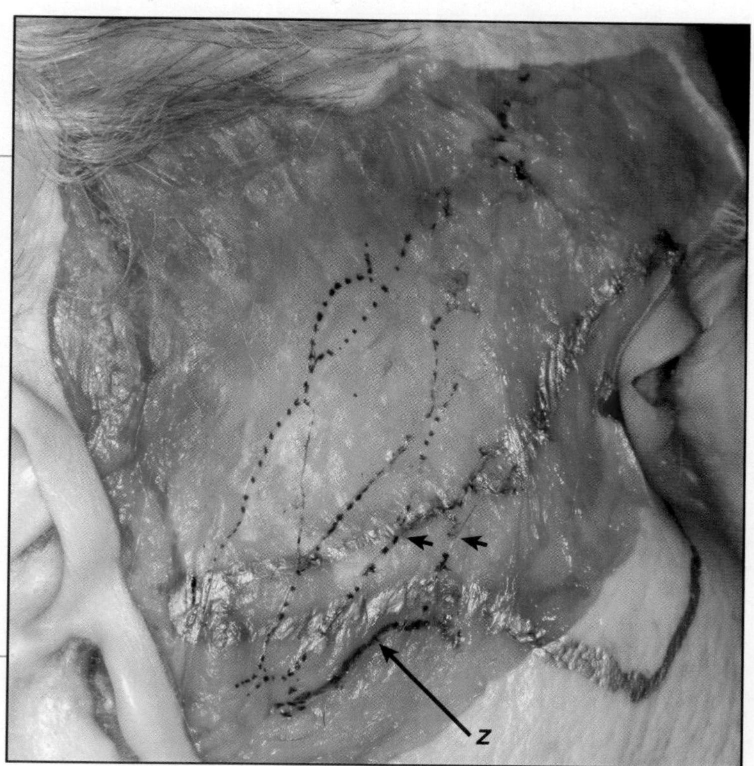

Figure 2.22

Same dissection with bone marked in silver for better understanding of the zygomatic branch (Z), which continues forward to be seen in further dissections.

There exists great overlap of nerves for the orbicularis oculi muscle. Three branches course upward to supply the frontalis and upper orbicularis muscles. From branch 3 as well as the zygomatic branch (Z), a branch goes to the lower orbicularis (*arrow*). The muscle area exactly lateral to the canthus would seem a safe area for excision of muscle for reduction of crow's feet. Also, note that the zygomatic branch to the lower eyelid usually runs deeply.

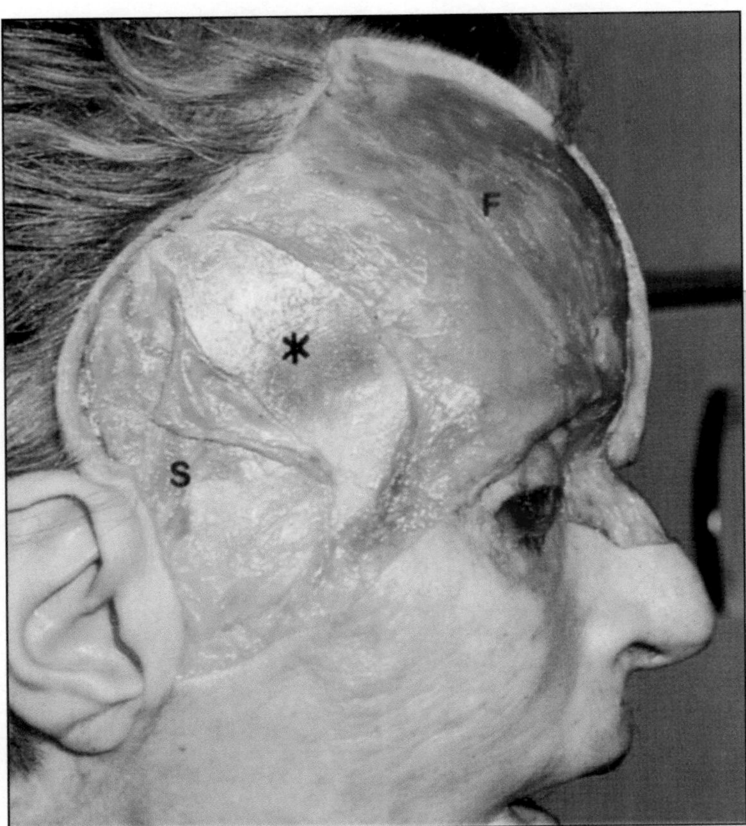

Figure 2.23

For the sake of completion, the temporal fascia is depicted here for clinical application in zygomatic arch elevation from above.

An incision is made between the frontalis muscle (F) and the superficial temporal fascial layer containing the superficial temporal vessels (S). Note the glistening temporalis fascia or deep temporal fascia which overlies the muscle (*).

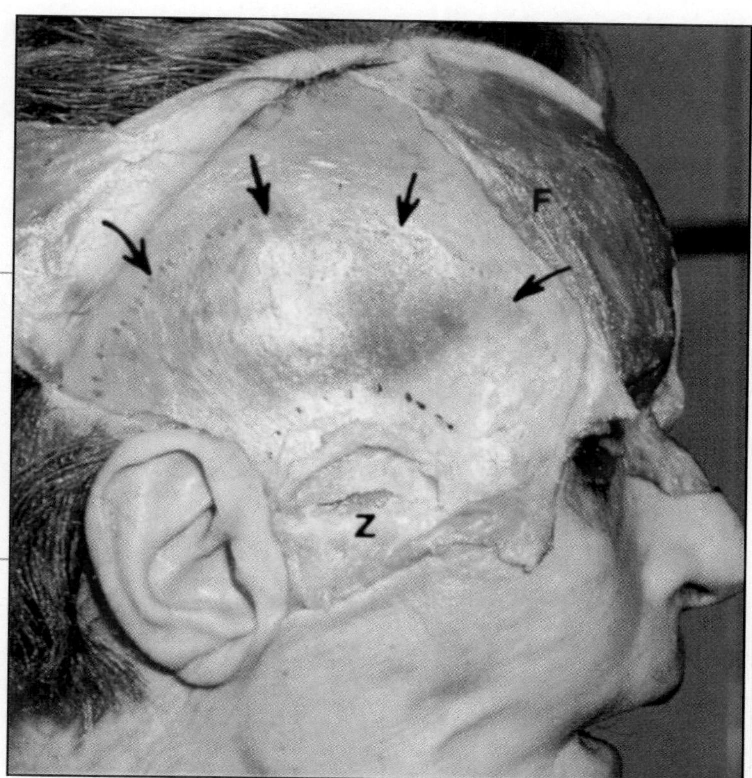

Figure 2.24

The superficial temporal fascia is retracted posteriorly. Note the cut edge of frontalis muscle (F). The small arrows outline the superior temporal line, where the temporalis fascia begins. The temporalis muscle lies below this line. The dotted line denotes the point at which the temporalis fascia splits prior to enveloping the zygomatic arch (Z).

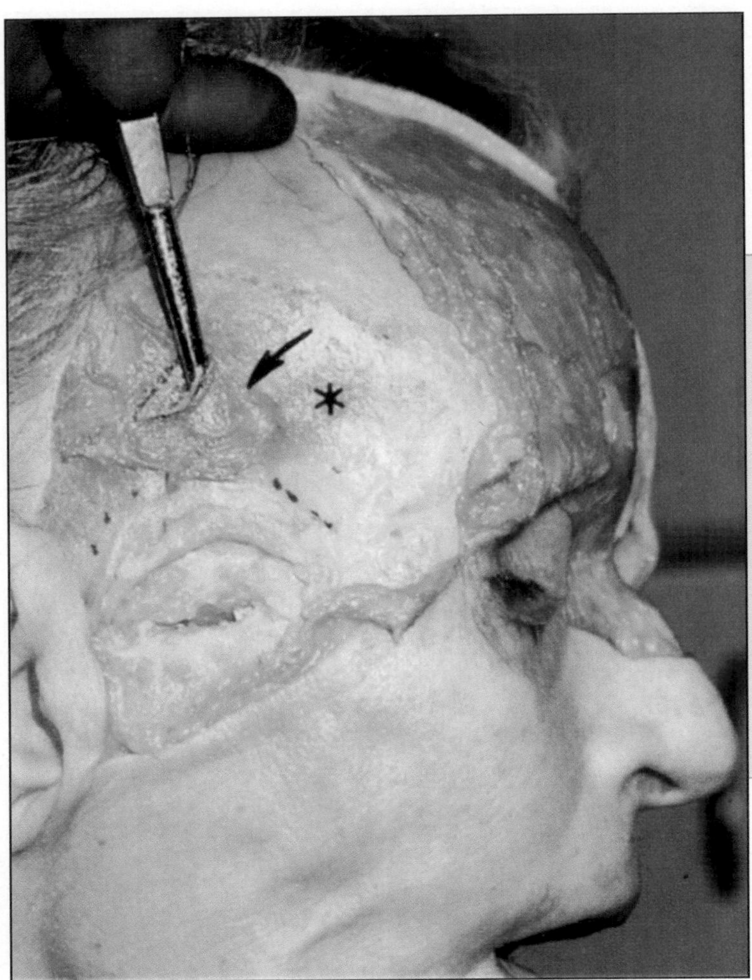

Figure 2.25

It is important to understand the relationship of the superficial and deep layers of the temporal fascia to the zygomatic arch when reducing fractures. In order to elevate a fractured zygomatic bone or its arch, the elevator must be placed beneath both layers above the point of fusion at which the deeper layer splits (*dotted*). This allows access to the medial aspect of the bone. In this dissection, a small remnant of superficial temporal fascia (*arrow*) has been preserved overlying the deep temporalis fascia (*). The elevator pierces both layers to lie on the surface of the temporalis muscle. Passage inferiorly provides access to the medial zygoma (Gillies maneuver).

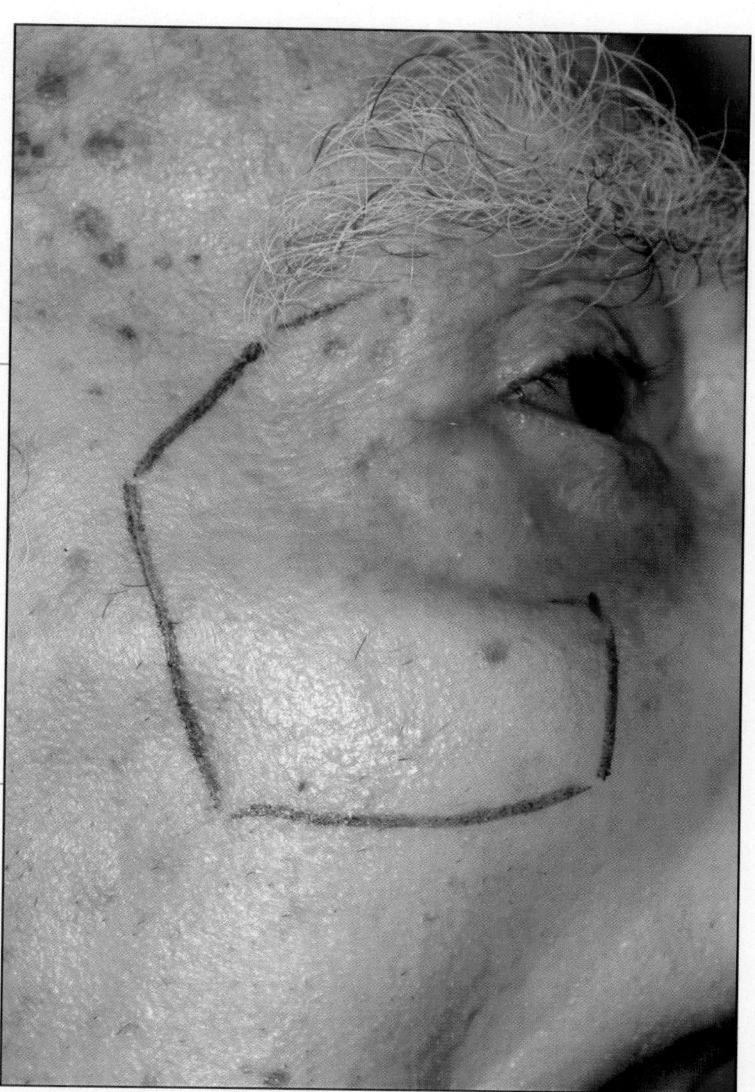

A

Figure 2.26A

Purple denotes the basic dissection zone and beyond. (We will start from above downward, then from below upward.)

Inferolateral zone: many of the newer procedures, especially subSMAS dissections and deep plane face lift methods require a thorough understanding of this zone. The plan of exposure will start first from above downward, demonstrating the orbital retaining ligaments (ORL), the insertion of the orbicularis oculi medially, the zygomaticus muscles and structures medial to that.

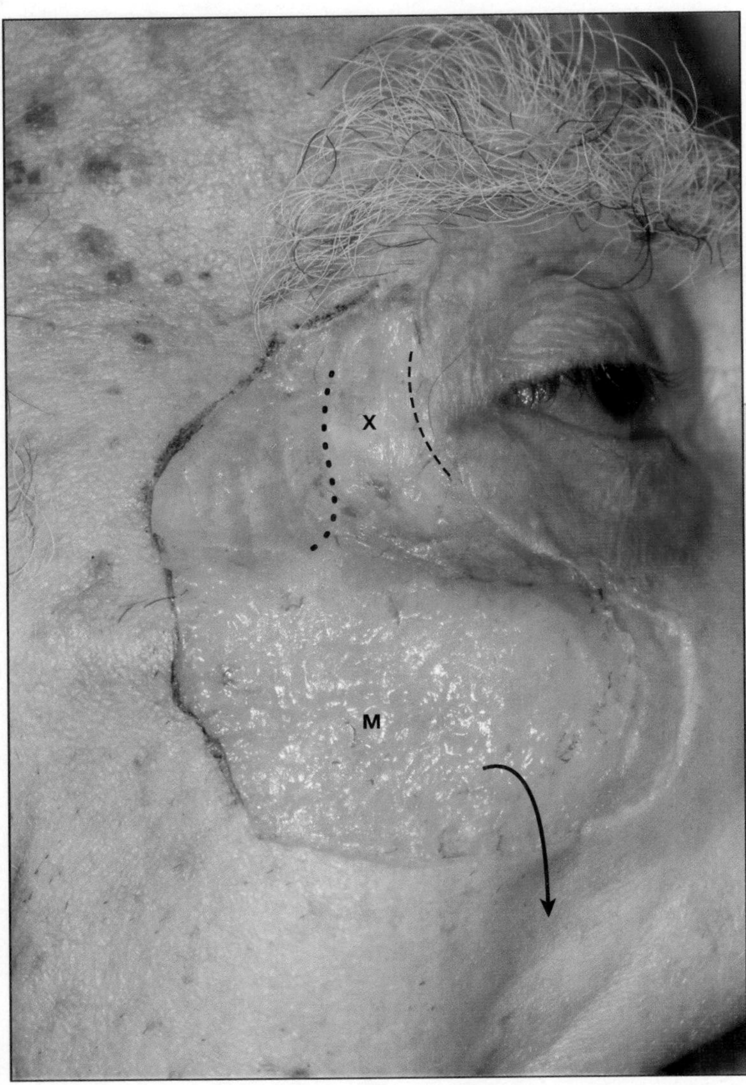

Figure 2.26B

Skin only removed; malar fat pad (M) is noted. The lateral orbital rim (X) is dashed at front and posterior borders. The orbicularis fibers are very thin in area X, i.e., over the rim, but you can see that the orbicularis ring extends far beyond the rim laterally. As the arrow shows the malar fat pad alone will now be dissected off the underlying orbicularis oculi (orbital part) and the zygomaticus major.

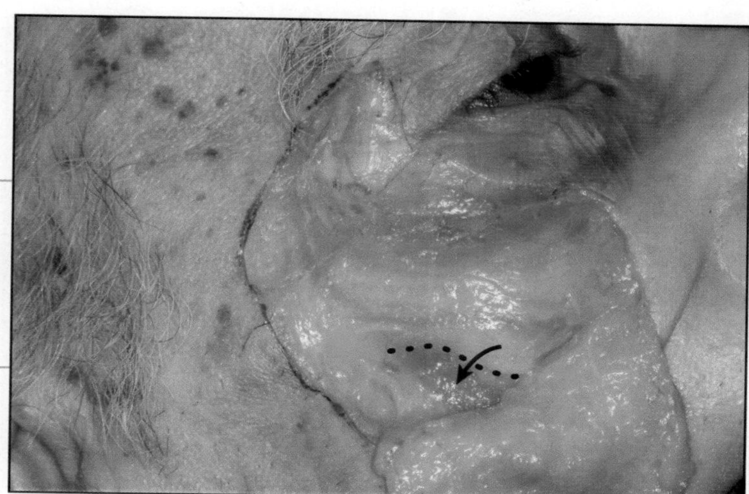

Figure 2.27

Malar fat pad dissected off orbicularis from above. Note that the orbital part of the orbicularis becomes thinned out and interspersed with fat. The arrow points to the upper part of the zygomaticus major.

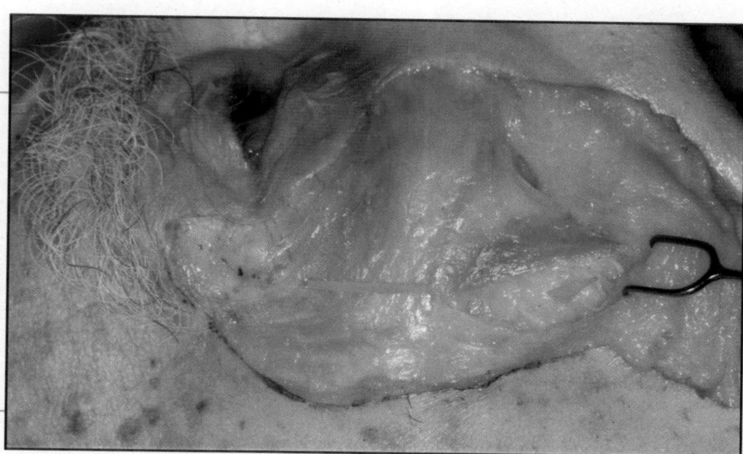

Figure 2.28

With downward traction on the malar fat pad, the zygomatic major muscle becomes exposed. The red dart shows the zygomatic branch of VII to this muscle. The red vertical paper shows that the muscle usually begins near a vertical line dropped from the lateral edge of the lateral orbital rim. This line might be drawn on the face when deep SMAS dissections are performed.

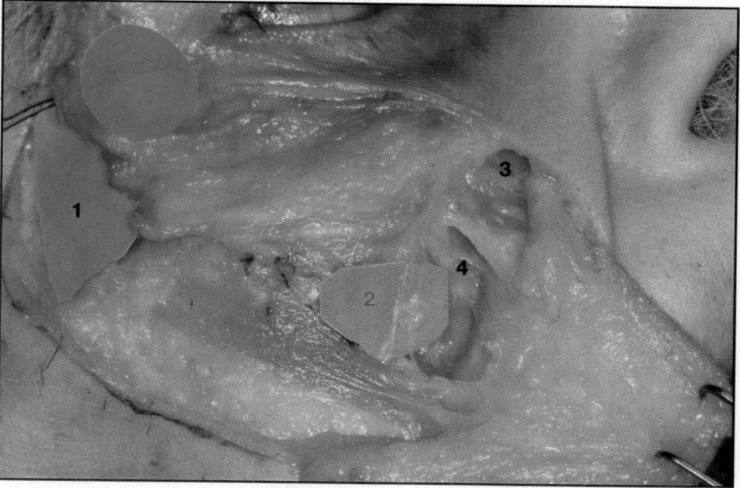

Figure 2.29

Green upper (1) lies along upper arch and posterior lateral orbital rim over the temporal fossa. Green lower paper (2) is below zygomatic branches that continue forward to supply the orbicularis oculi and beyond. The levator muscles (3) are noted, with the caninus muscle (4) below. The infraorbital foramen opens below the levator origin, which can be seen well in other dissections.

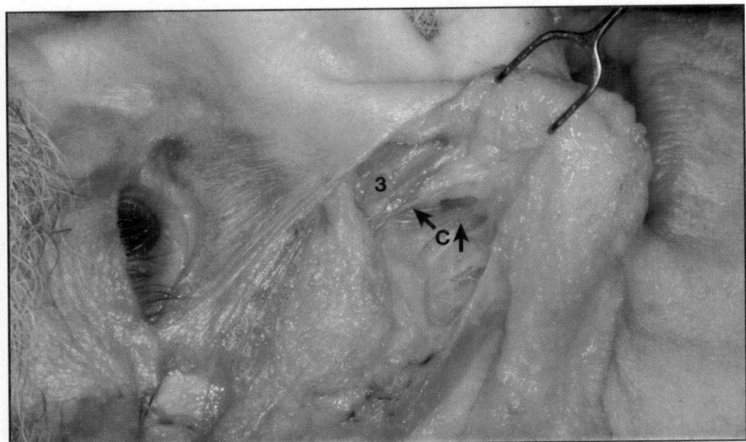

A

Figure 2.30A

Body from side. Below the levator muscles (3), an arrow points to a branch off the infraorbital nerve. The caninus muscle can be seen arising from the maxillary face (c) (*lower arrow*). The other upper arrow points to the infraorbital nerve, a lateral branch of which is obvious.

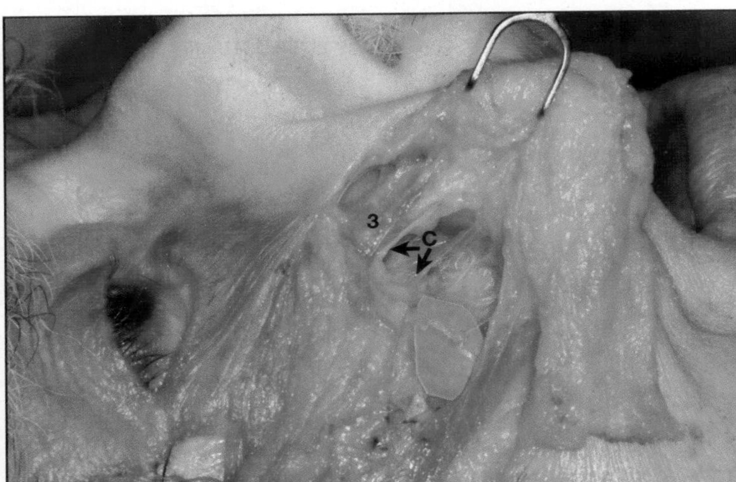

B

Figure 2.30B

Note the zygomatic branch over the green pad proceeding medially.

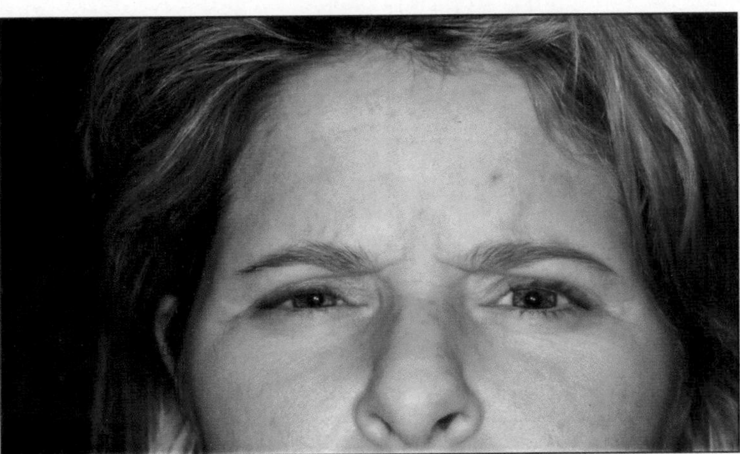

Figure 2.31

Local in vivo injection study. The subject is asked to "squinch" her brows maximally. The medial brows descend. Muscle bulk above the medial brow is caused by corrugator action. The medial brows are pulled down by the medial orbicularis oculi, depressor superulli, and the procerus muscles.

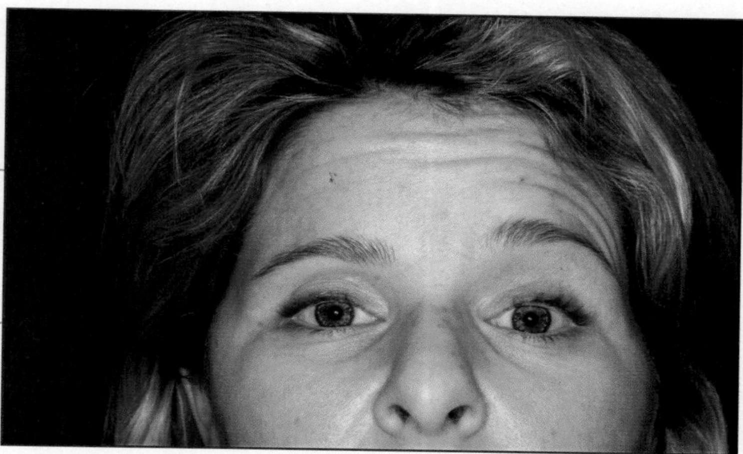

Figure 2.32

Anesthetic is placed over the zygomatic arch along the 0.8- to 3.5-cm path of the frontal branch as noted previously. The right frontalis cannot elevate the brow.

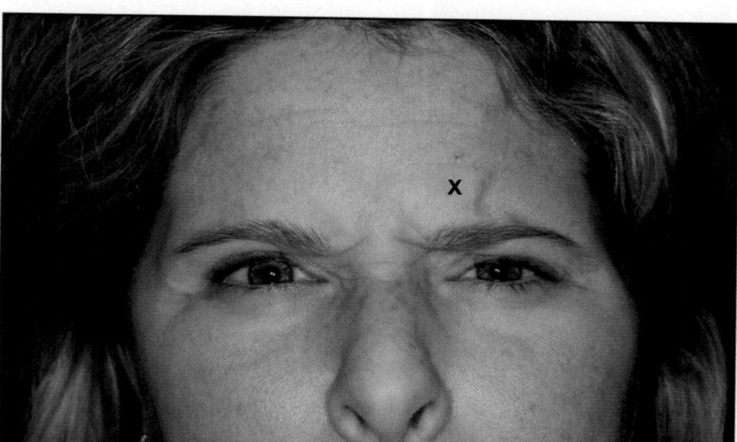

Figure 2.33

On maximum "squinch," the right medial brow *still* depresses. Corrugator bulk is noted on the left (X) but not on the right. It is possible that the procerus also is here. Its newer supply may also be infact.

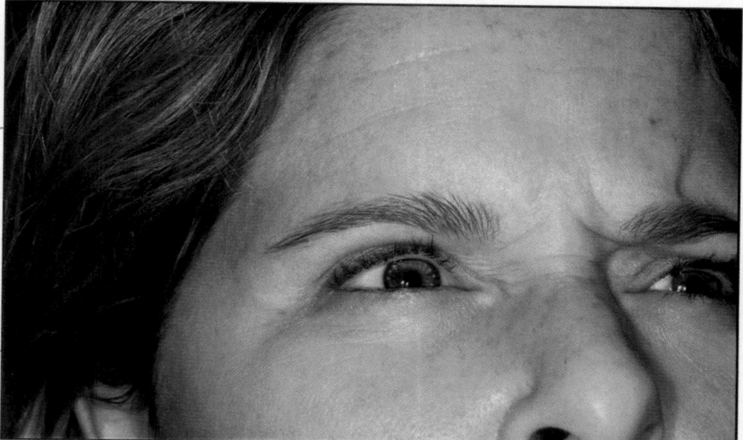

Figure 2.34

Close-up. The medial orbicularis oculi and depressor supercilii cause the brow to move down, and oblique wrinkles are made in the hollow. This means that obliteration of the nerves to the corrugator will not prevent medial brow descension.

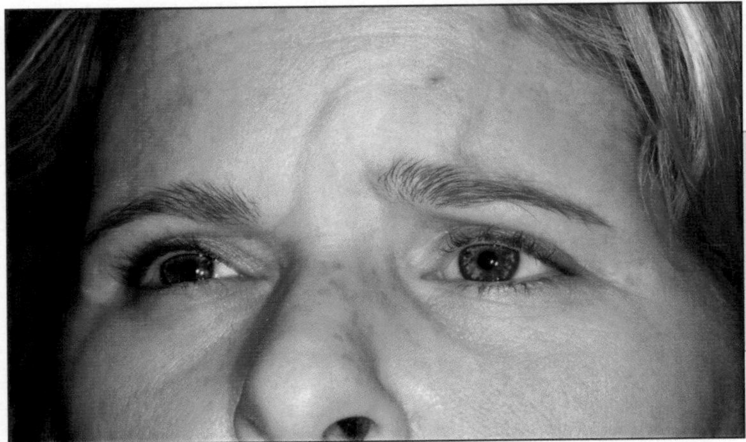

Figure 2.35

The zygomatic branches are blocked below the arch and behind the zygomaticus major on the left. Following zygomatic branch block, the corrugator on the left can still work but the medial brow does not descend. The procerus also seems not to work.

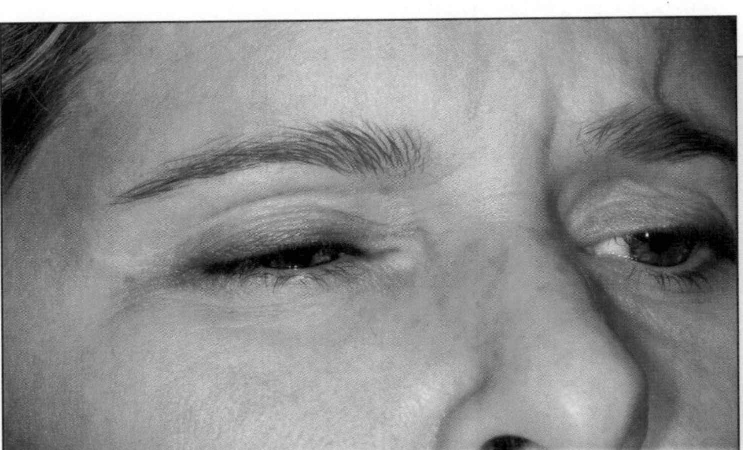

Figure 2.36

On the right side, the corrugator does not work and the medial brow does descend.

Explanation: The zygomatic branch must continue its course medially and over the medial canthus to supply the medial orbicularis oculi and depressor supercilii. Corrugator removal alone or nerve removal alone will not prevent brow descension. More muscle removal will be required. The procerus may also receive supply from the zygomatic branch, but the author is not absolutely sure.

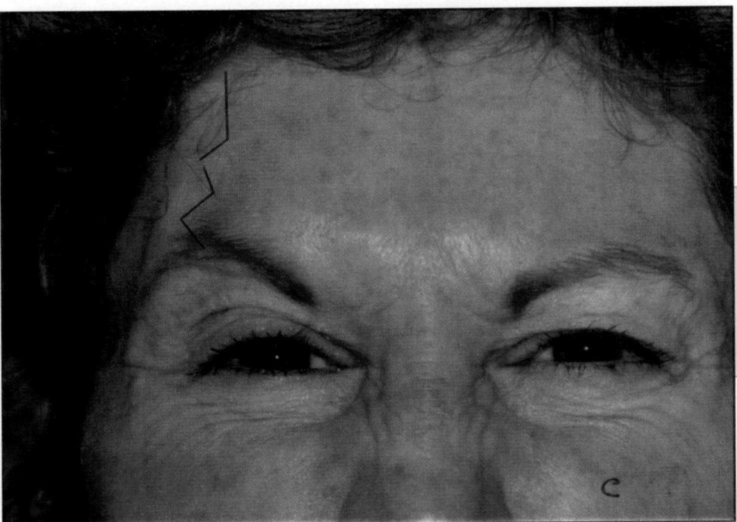

Figure 2.37

A 54-year-old woman with a scar (*black*) as noted s/p motor vehicle accident serves as a validating study. Note: depressors of medial brow work, but the ipsilateral corrugator is not functioning.

Figure 2.38

In this live demonstration the sentinal vein is clearly visible as it comes out of the deep temporal fascia. Although this is supposed to be a landmark for the surgeon, i.e., that the frontal branches are in a centimeter circle around the entrance into the overlying tissue, it is more just a clinical entity that the surgeon should recognize. In practice, the author has noted that transection of this vessel does lead to more swelling in that area in the postoperative period, but that seems to be the only significance from the surgeon's perspective.

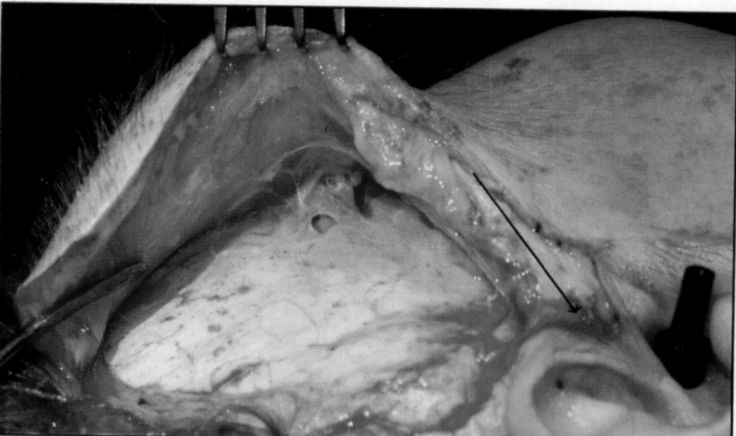

CHAPTER 3

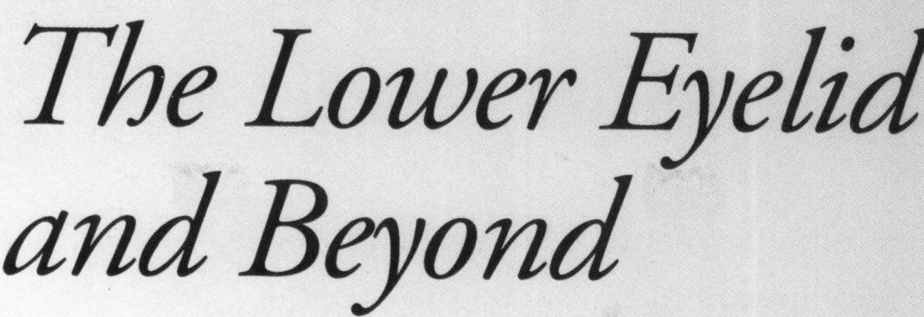

The Lower Eyelid and Beyond

The earlier edition treated the eyelids together, but here the dissections go beyond that to expose those structures in separate zones. This chapter exposes the lower eyelid inferolateral zone.

These studies extend downward to expose the suborbicularis oculi fat (SOOF), orbital retaining ligaments (ORL), and the zygomatic/elevator muscles. Ligaments and nerves are emphasized, key for performing sub-superficial musculo-aponeurotic system dissections. The dissection continues laterally and upward to expose the fascia below the lateral orbicularis muscles. This lateral orbital thickening (LOT), is triangular with the apex laterally placed. The size of this fascial area decreases with age.

Inferior and Lateral to the Orbital Rim

1 The orbicularis oculi attaches directly to the inferior orbital rim from the anterior lacrimal crest to the medial limbus of the cornea. Thus, to approach the medial SOOF, you must transect this muscle at the bony rim. As the patient ages, some of the more lateral muscle attachment may pull away from the rim as the check droops.

1a If you continue dissection medially through the orbicularis oculi, the next key structure you would approach is the levator labii superioris alaeque nasi, under which resides the infraorbital foramen with its nerve and vessels.

2 Laterally, the orbital septum attaches along the rim and a little beyond, but the orbicularis muscle attaches to the rim indirectly here via multiple ligaments. Thus, to expose the SOOF, here these ligaments (ORL) need to be transected. These are the orbital retaining ligaments (ORL).

3 These retaining ligaments, which go from the periosteum to the suborbicularis fascia, continue laterally and upward to the lateral orbital rim.

3a The zygomaticofacial nerves exit the bone inferior to these ligaments to supply sensation over the cheek prominence and inferiorly. The sensory area can be represented by an inverted triangle with the apex downward.

3b These ORLs continue around and upward in continuity with the suborbicularis fascia below the orbicularis muscle laterally. The "lateral orbital thickening" as noted LOT varies in size; older bodies seem to have less.

3c If the ORLs are released below the inferior orbital rim and laterally (i.e., the LOT as well), the orbicularis connections with the lower lid to bone will be severed, and this will allow movement of the entire lid. Thus, redraping of the pretarsal and preseptal orbicularis would require release of the ligaments. With medial release of rim attachments the orbicularis oculi can be fully redraped if necessary.

4 A thick, subcutaneous malar fat pad overlies the cheek bone from the rim downward. The fat pad covers the lower orbital fibers of the orbicularis oculi, which extend considerably over the cheek. Fibers are interspersed with fat.

5 If by dissection the orbicularis oculi muscle and fascia are elevated from below after malar fat pad is swept down, these orbital retaining ligaments can be approached from below. This area up to the ligaments has been dubbed the "prezygomatic space."

6 By elevating the lower orbicularis muscle and fascia upward, the zygomaticus major muscle fibers become exposed. The lateral zygomaticus fibers begin on a plumb line dropped down a little laterally to the lateral part of the lateral orbital rim. (Remember this!)

7 The zygomatic branch of cranial nerve VII innervates the zygomaticus muscles and continues onward to innervate the lower orbicularis oculi, levator muscles, and even the *upper lid* depressor supercilii and medial orbicularis oculi (and perhaps the procerus).

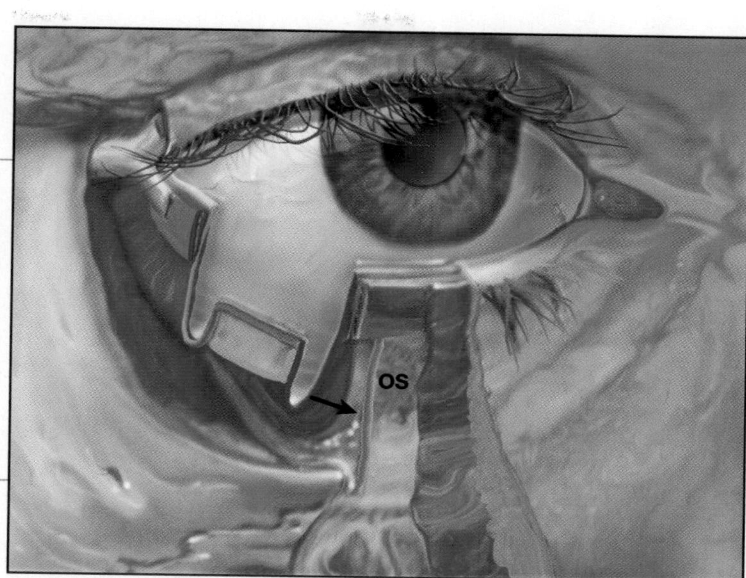

Figure 3.1

The anterior lamella of the lower lid consists of skin and underlying muscle. Note the cut edge of the orbital septum (OS), which meets at the junction of periosteum and periorbita, the arcus marginalis (*lower arrow*). The upper arrow denotes the capsulopalpebral fascia, an extension of the inferior rectus muscle that acts to lower the eyelid in unison with the globe during downward gaze.

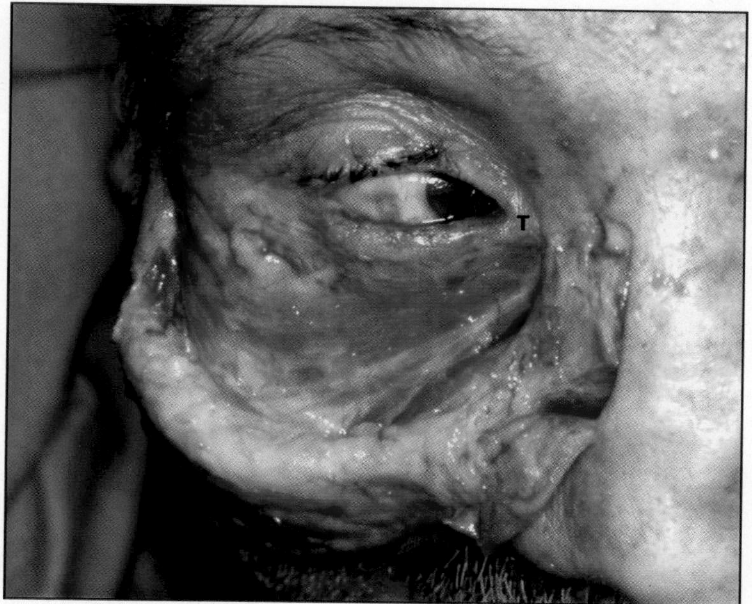

Figure 3.2

The skin and malar fat pad of the lower eyelid are retracted inferiorly, exposing the orbicularis oculi muscle. Note the horizontal orientation of the blood supply in the upper portion of the muscle. These represent branches of the inferior medial and lateral palpebral branches derived from the infratrochlear and lacrimal arteries, respectively. The arterial supply courses in a submuscular plane and receives anastomosing twigs from the angular, infraorbital, transverse facial, and zygomaticofacial vessels.

Note that the orbicularis oculi muscle originates from the medial canthal tendon (T) and from the lower medial orbital margin. The orbicularis fibers sweep temporally, covering the origins of the elevators of the upper lip and nasal ala. They extend across the cheek to overlie the anterior part of the temporalis fascia. The upper orbicularis is supplied by the temporal branch of cranial nerve VII with some small twigs off the zygomatic branch. Lymphatic drainage from the lateral side is into the preauricular and parotid nodes. The medial side drains into the submandibular regional nodes.

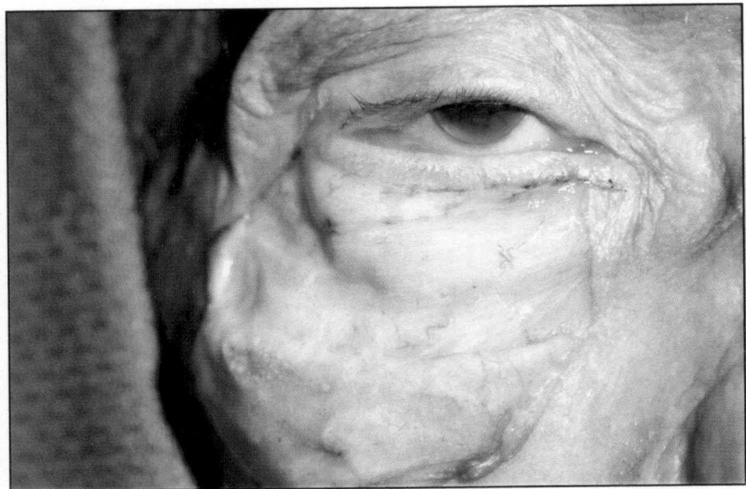

Figure 3.3

Muscle thickness varies from person to person. In this dissection, the orbital septum and fat are visible in spite of "skin-only" removal. The muscle, therefore, is quite thin, easily explaining how scant muscle, bony hypoplasia ("negative vector"), and thin septum would predispose to bulging fat, as well as a possible ptotic lid.

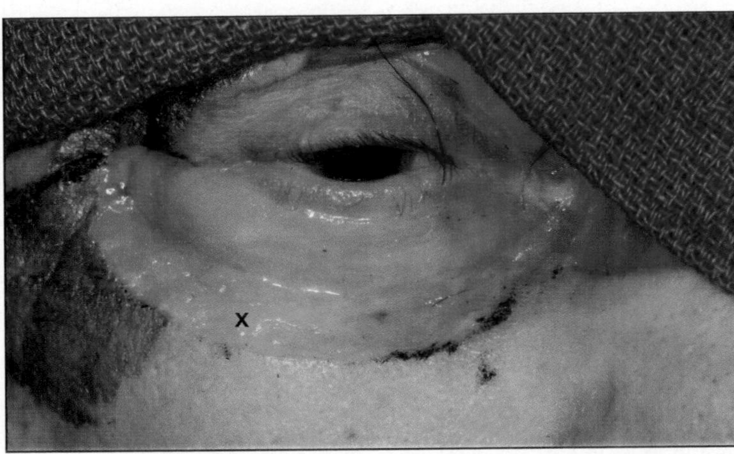

Figure 3.4

In this younger specimen, the orbicularis muscle (pretarsal and preseptal portions) covers the orbital septum evenly. Note the thick malar fat pad (X) under the cheek skin.

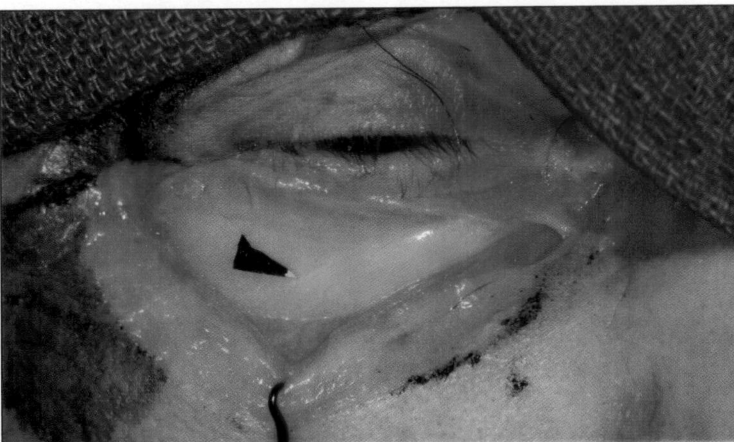

Figure 3.5

A cut-through muscle with hook retraction inferiorly exposes the orbital septum here with fat behind it. The dart points to the arcuate ligament, which separates the lateral and middle fat pads.

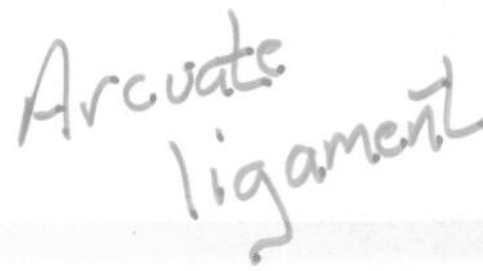

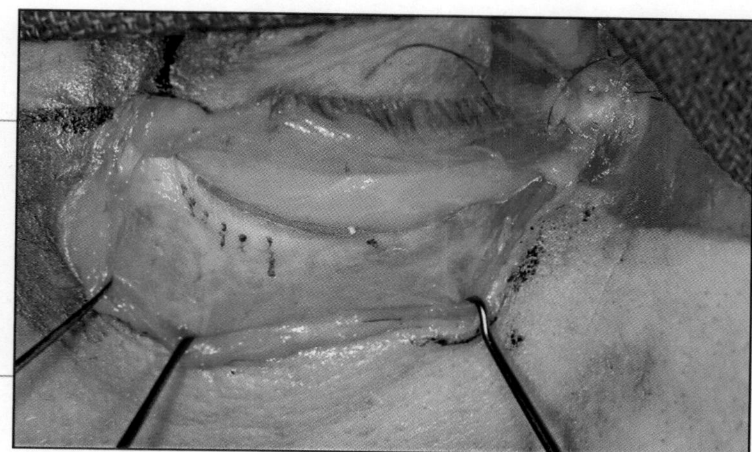

Figure 3.6

The blue strip marks the inferior orbital rim at the arcus marginalis. Note that the orbicularis fibers are attached to the rim along the medial half at least. The short blue vertical lines are ligamentous attachments from the rim to the orbicularis underside. These ligaments have been called orbital retaining ligaments (ORLs).

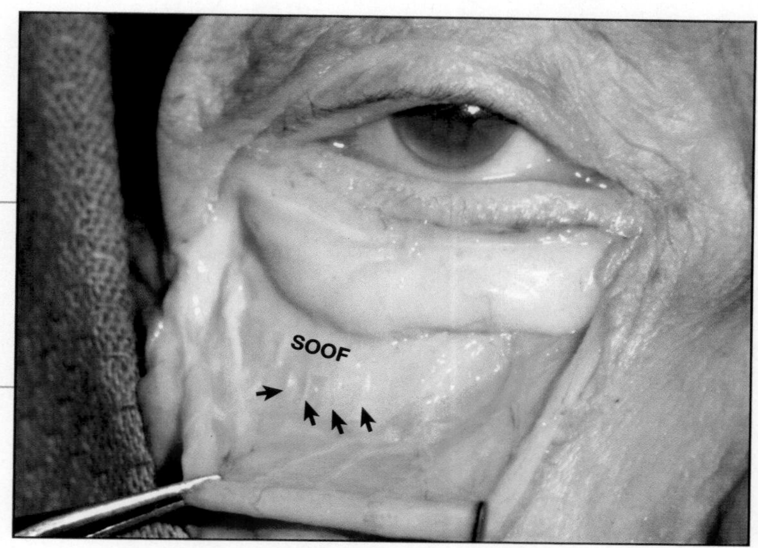

Figure 3.7

The ligaments are visible here and marked (*arrow*). The suborbicularis oculi fat (SOOF) over the bone is exposed with transection of these ligaments. The zygomaticofacial nerves are always inferior to them.

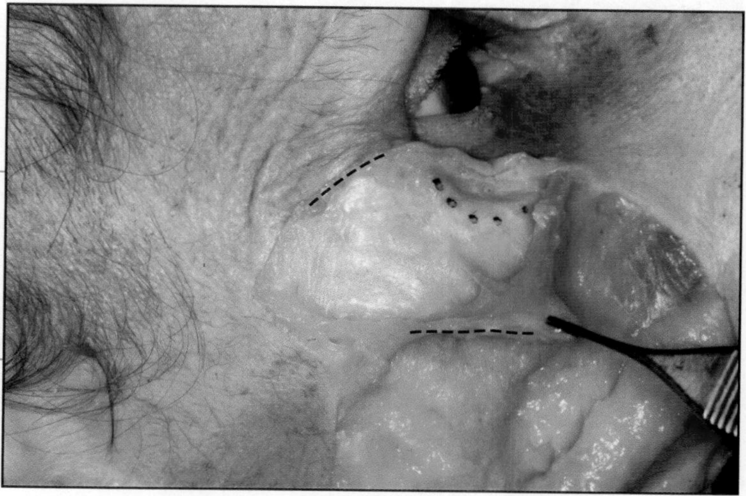

Figure 3.8

Lateral view: Black dots are placed along the orbital rim. The orbicularis is grasped with forceps. Note the ligaments to the bone and the SOOF below the black dots. The dashed lines shows where the orbicularis oculi was transected.

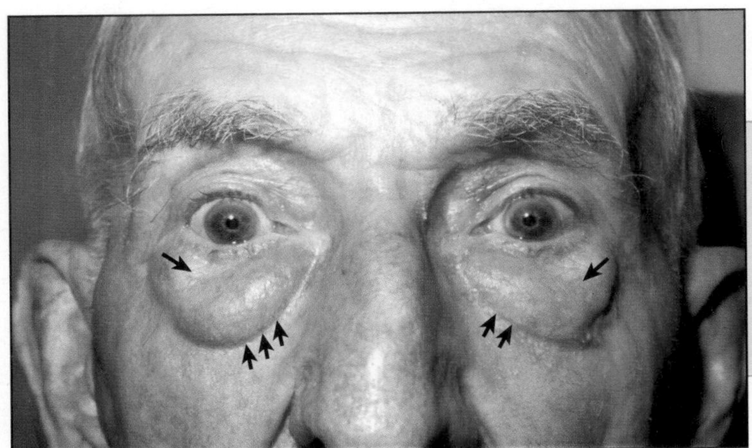

Figure 3.9A

The arcuate ligament notches the fat bilaterally (*arrows*). The fat descension over the rim is allowed by a thin orbital septum, which occurs with age. The ORLs (*dots*) hold the lateral fat over the rim from going lower. The lateral part of the orbicularis attachment to the rim has probably detached at the lower arrows.

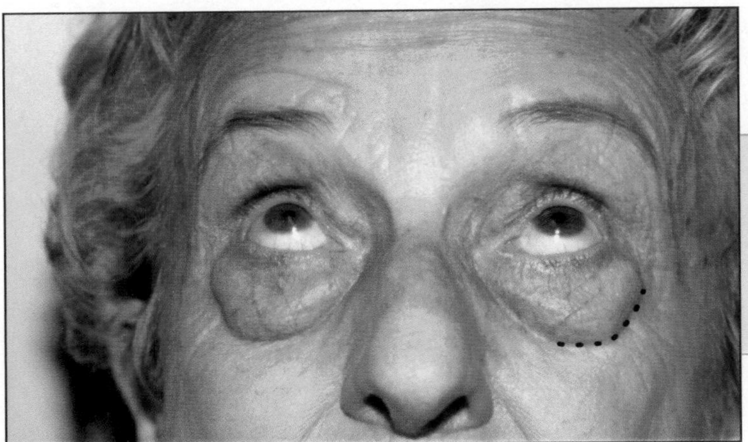

B

Figure 3.9B

With upgaze the fat prolapse becomes more obvious. The dots show how far the fat has descended beyond and below the rim. The ORLs must have been pushed down to allow this as well the orbicularis attachment was likely pushed away along the central rim.

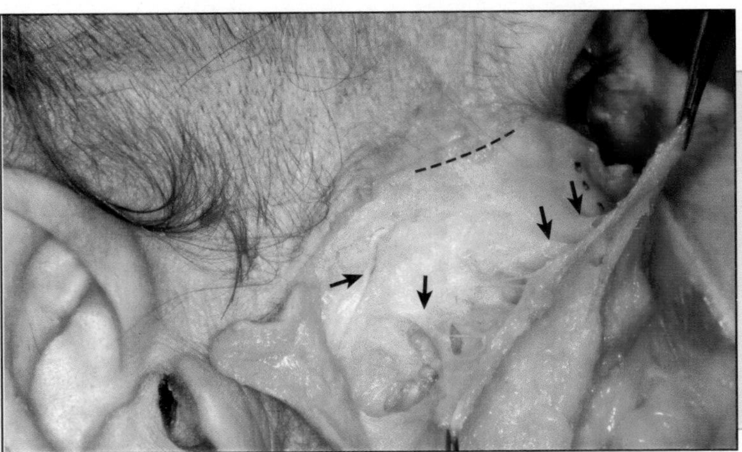

Figure 3.10

Dotted lines: The orbicularis oculi was cut transversely just below the lateral canthal region and retracted downward (*dashes*). Two sets of ligaments are now visible. While holding the orbicularis oculi outward, the orbital retaining ligaments are seen (*upper arrows*) and zygomaticocutaneous ligaments are noted below the zygomatic arch (*lower arrow*). A frontal nerve branch has a small blue streak placed on it (*arrow closest to ear*).

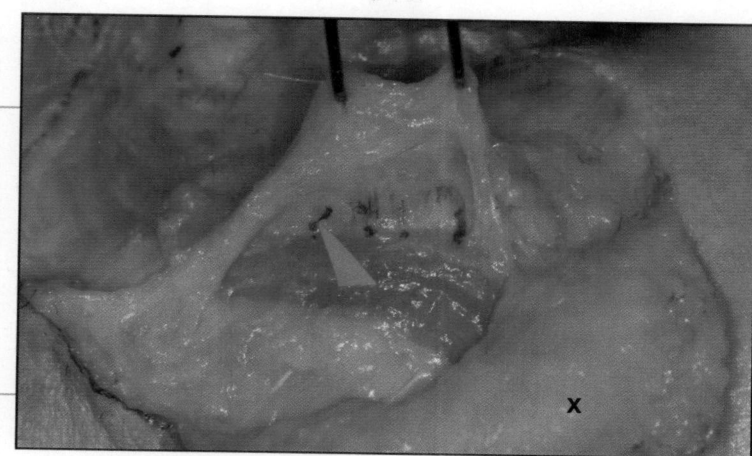

Figure 3.11

The dissection will now shift. The orbicularis oculi will be lifted from below. The malar fat pad, of course, has already been retracted downward (X). The lower orbicularis muscle and fat and the underlying fascia are elevated with a double hook, and the ORLs (*blue marks and red dart*) are noted. The zygomaticus major muscle is below the dart.

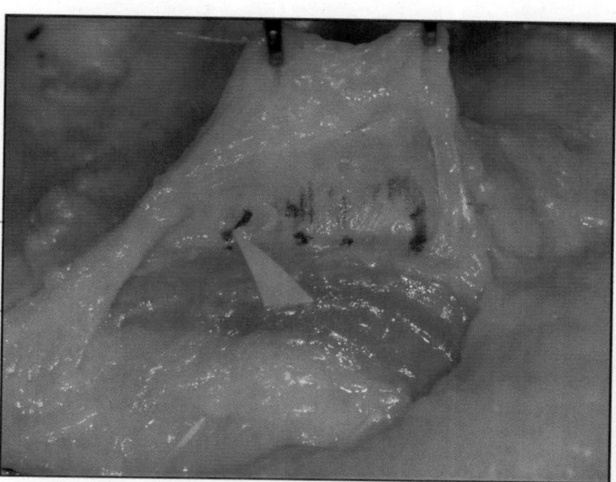

Figure 3.12

The orbicularis is not cut; rather, it is lifted with its underlying fascia from the outer edges.

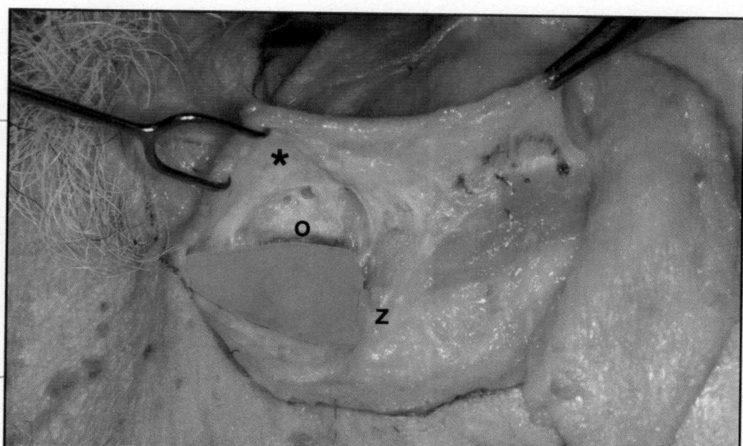

Figure 3.13

A green sheet is placed along the bones in the temporal fossa. The orbital rim (O) and zygomatic arch (Z) are noted. The thick fascia, the LOT (*), is seen under the orbicularis muscle with attachments to the rim. The orbital retaining ligaments are clearly seen at the lower orbicularis attachment to bone.

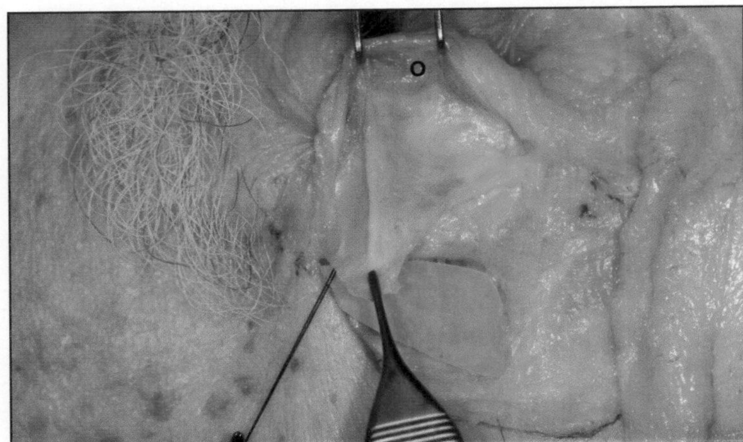

Figure 3.14

A black suture has been placed around the lateral canthal tendon (not seen yet). The fascia (LOT) is being separated from the orbicularis oculi muscles above it (O).

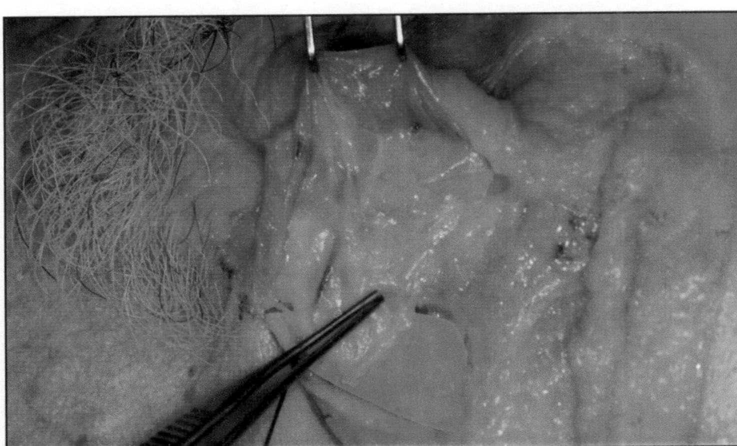

Figure 3.15

As the dissection proceeds, one can see the lateral fat pad (*red dart*) of the lower lid. The silk suture outline is noted on course to the deep lateral canthal tendon as it inserts onto Whitnall's tubercle inside the rim.

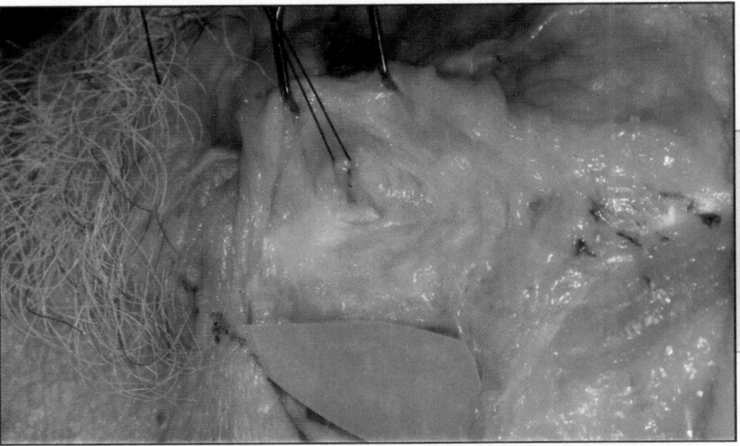

Figure 3.16

Flipping the orbital thickening back upward, some of the attachments to the rim are cut, so you can see the suture around the lateral canthal tendon (*blue line*) prior to its insertions into Whitnall's tubercle, the bony bump inside the rim.

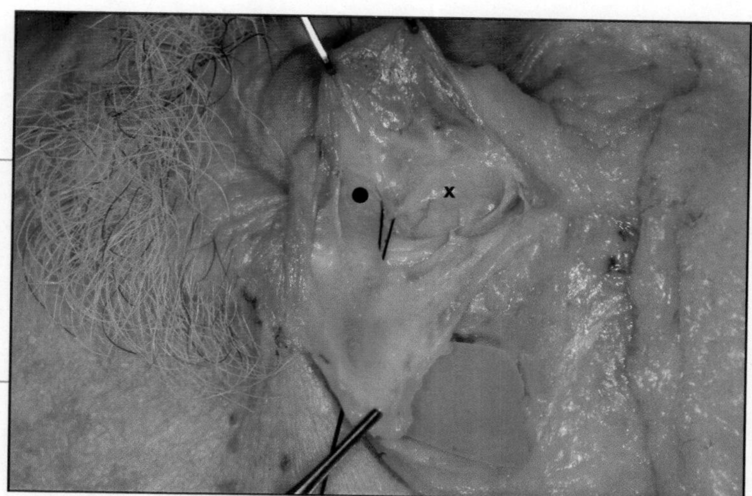

Figure 3.17

Flipping the LOT back over, the size of the lateral orbital thickening is better seen. The lower lateral fat pad is visible (X). The suture to the tendons is seen passing under the thickening. Even some of the upper lateral fat pad is visible (•).

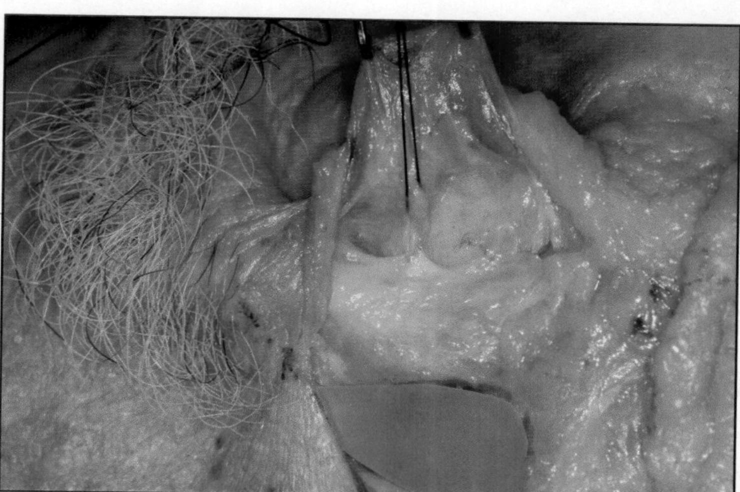

Figure 3.18

The LOT has been removed to expose the periosteum on the rim. The suture is pulling up the lateral canthal tendon.

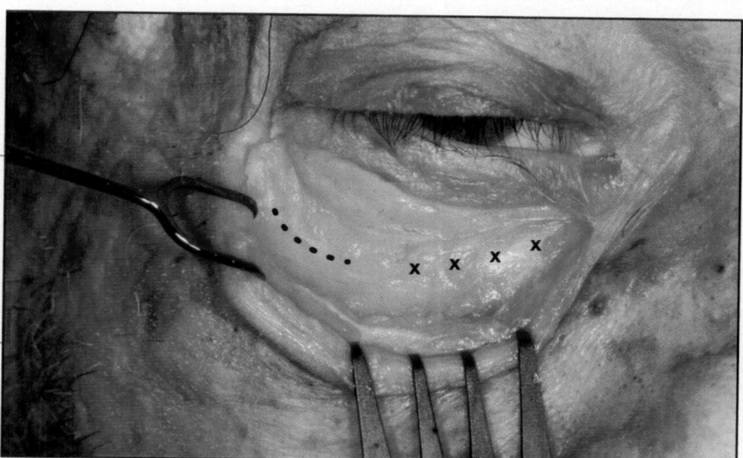

Figure 3.19

SOOF exposure and beyond: The orbicularis oculi is divided between pretarsal and preseptal parts. The attachments of the orbicularis to rim are cut at X's. The ORLs are cut below the lateral rim (*dots*).

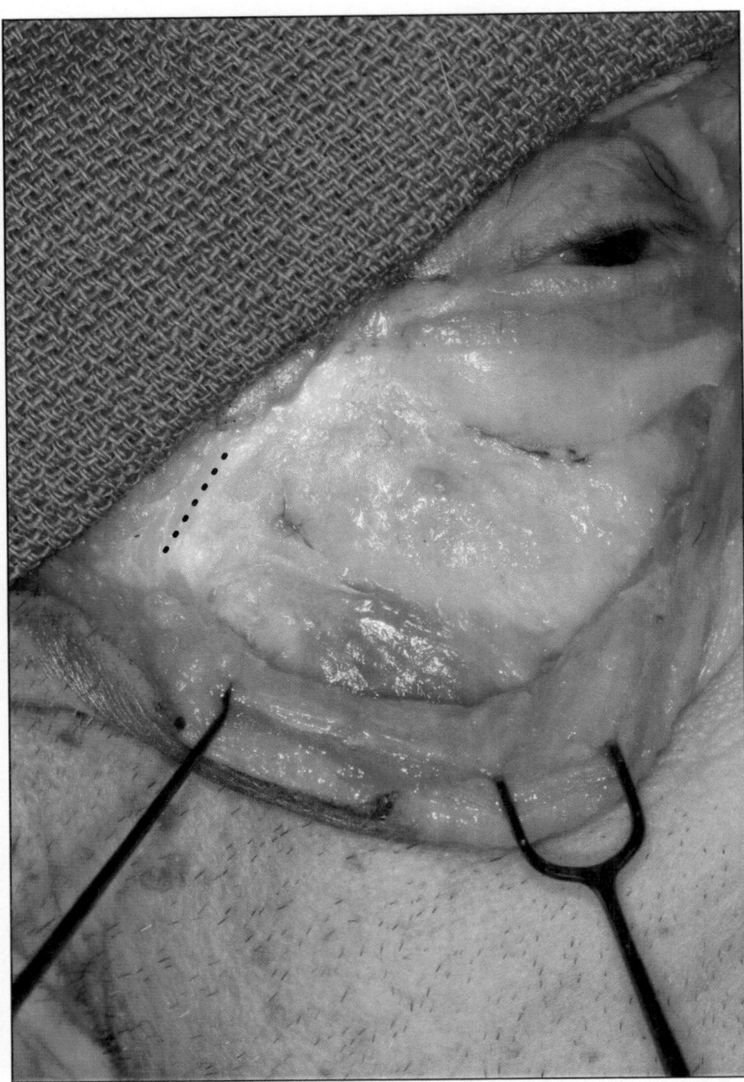

Figure 3.20

All the ORL of the malar area are cut. The orbicularis is transected laterally (*dots*). The muscle is retracted downward, further exposing the origin of the zygomaticus major with the SOOF above; the origin starts around a plumb line down from the lateral part of the lateral orbital rim.

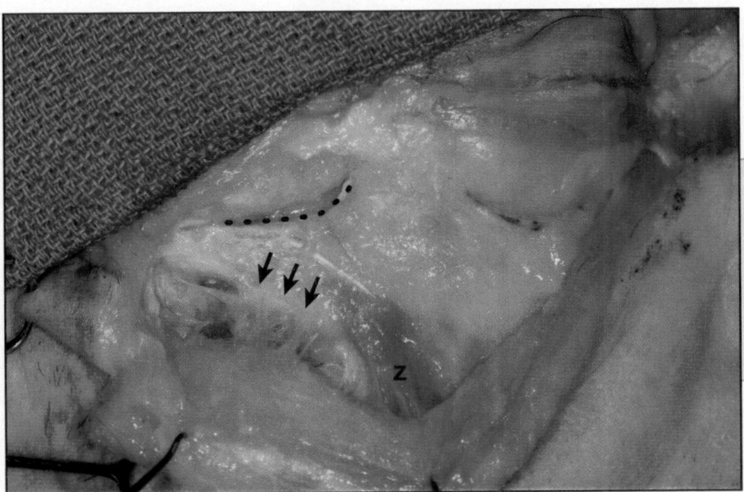

Figure 3.21

The fascia is cut along the 2-cm safe zone behind the rim to show the upper border of the zygomatic arch (*dotted*). Along the lower arch opposite the safe zone, but before the zygomaticus muscle (Z), the zygomatico-cutaneous ligaments are marked with arrows.

Figure 3.22

The upper and lower borders of the zygomatic arch are marked with silver. The nerve to the zygomaticus major is noted (*red dart*). A vertical line (*arrow*) dropped from just lateral to the lateral rim touches the lateral zygomatic major origin (O); with the ligaments cut and some fat removed, the fascia over the masseter fascia (M) and masseter muscle (M_2) are noted. The zygomatic branch of cranial nerve VII over the masseter fascia is noted (7), with its branch going into the zygomaticus major at the (*red dart*).

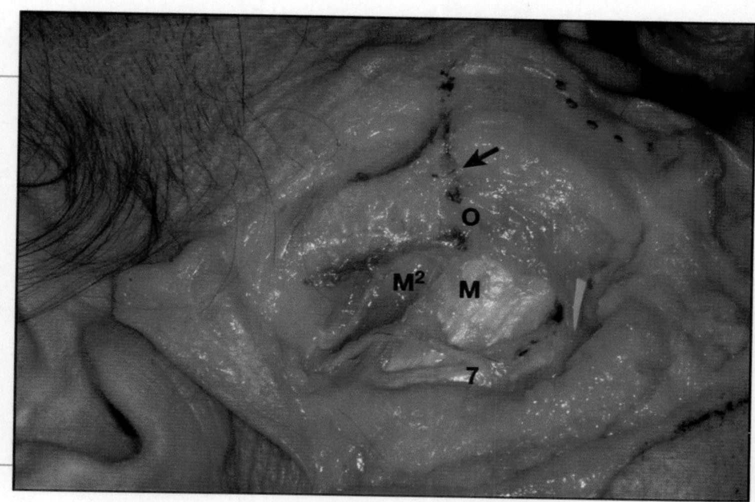

Figure 3.23

Moving medially: If the SOOF dissection is taken medially after the orbicularis is cut, the upper edge of the levator muscles is noted (*arrow*).

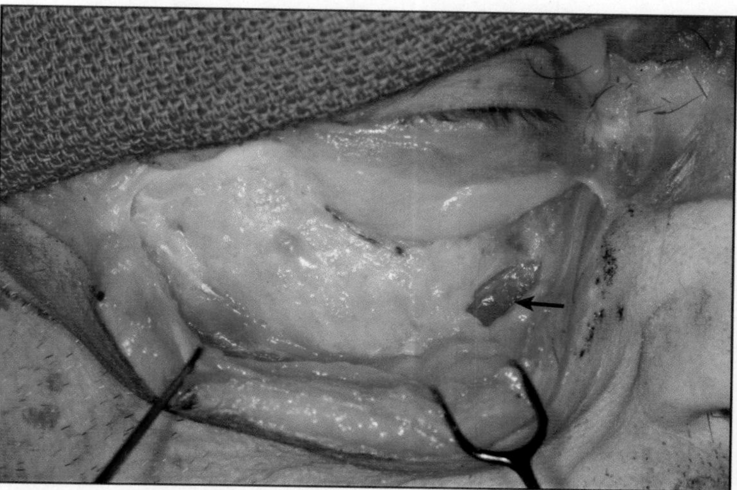

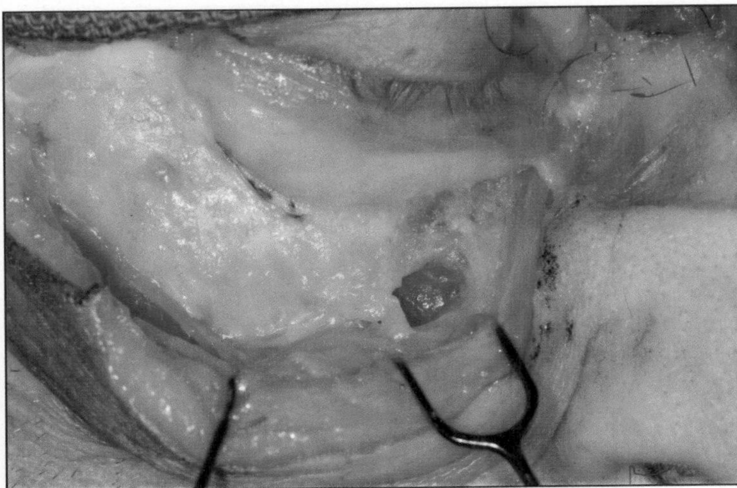

Figure 3.24

Close-up from above as in a clinical case.

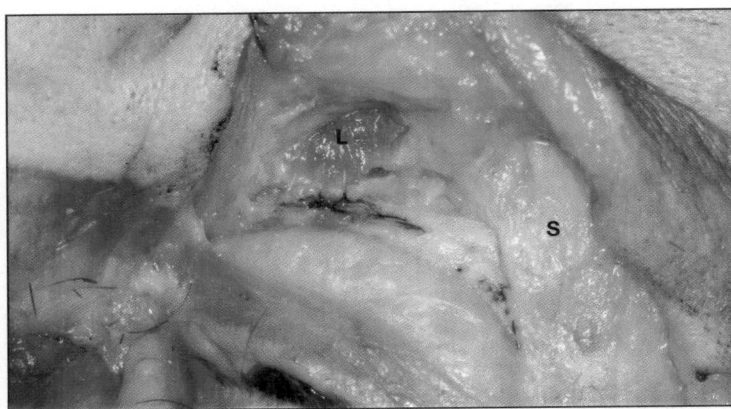

Figure 3.25

The medial purple line shows where the orbicularis oculi was removed from the rim. At this juncture the levator labii origin (L) is cut and the SOOF is elevated subperiosteally (S).

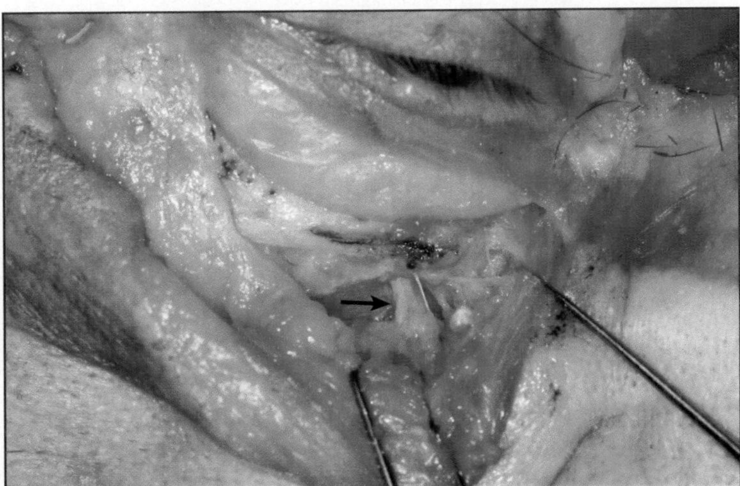

Figure 3.26

From the front the hook laterally pulls the SOOF forward with the periosteum. The levator labii now fully transected has been pulled away with the medial hook. The infraorbital nerve branches (*arrow*) are clearly visible about 7 mm from the rim in this case.

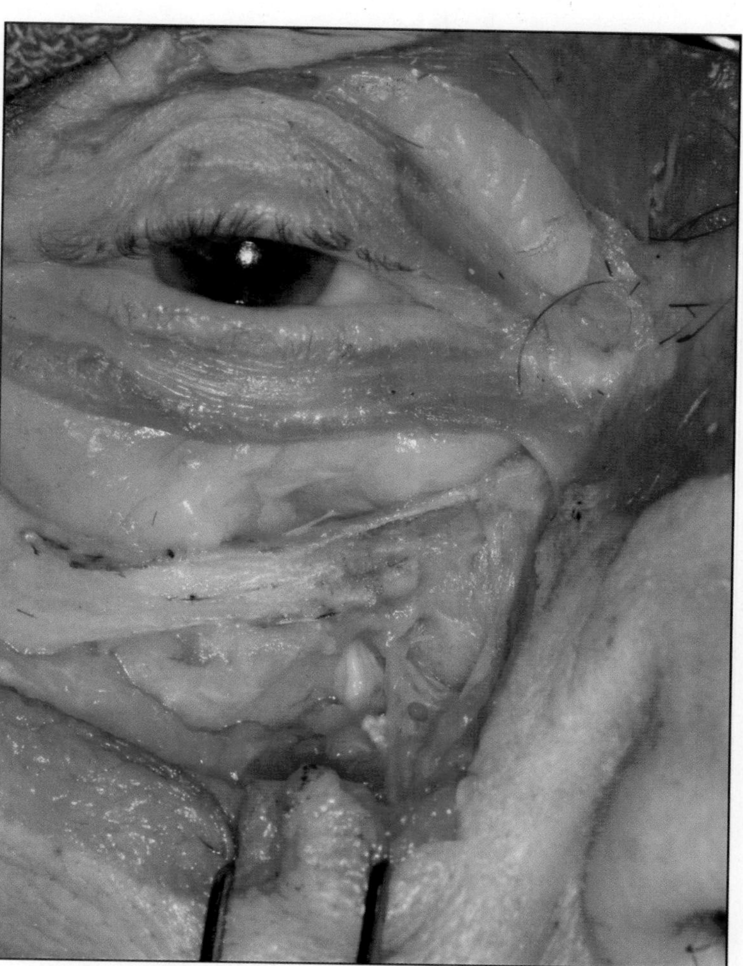

Figure 3.27

Measuring from the anterior nasal spine (ANS) as midline (ML), the infraorbital foramen is 2.4 to 2.7 cm from midline in females and 2.7 to 3.0 cm from ML in males. The rim-to-foramen distance in females is 5.5 to 6 mm; in males, it is 6.8 to 7.4 mm.

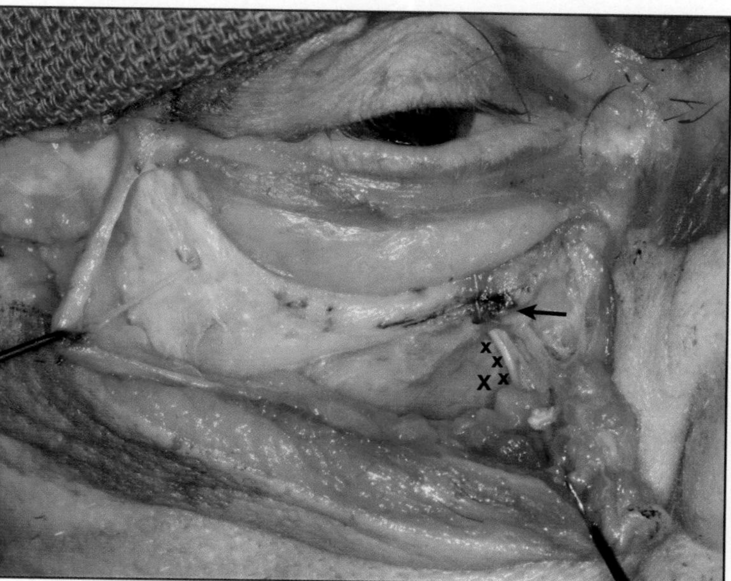

Figure 3.28

To reiterate: Medially, the orbicularis oculi is attached to the rim for 50% or more, then a layer of fat, then the levator labii superior is the origin of which is noted by the thicker purple line (*arrow*). Then the nerve and, below that, the caninus muscle (Xs) below the nerve.

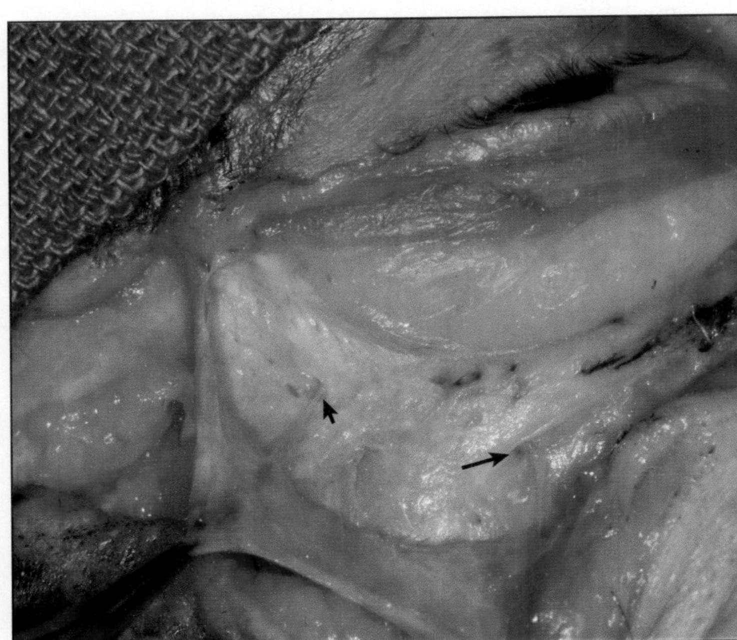

Figure 3.29

Subperiosteal dissection. In this specimen, two zygomaticofacial nerves exit near the junction of the inferior and lateral rims (*arrows*). A cheek implant dissection here obviously might transect these, and thus the malar region and below would be numb for a while.

CHAPTER 4

ROOF and Beyond (Superolateral Zone)

The "ROOF"—Retro-orbicularis oculi fat

1. Below the superolateral orbicularis oculi (preseptal and orbital part) and suborbicularis fascia, but above the orbital septum, the retro-orbicularis oculi fat (ROOF) pad extends from beyond the mid-supraorbital rim to beyond the lateral orbital rim.

2. This fat pad contributes to fullness in the upper lid and may require removal or reduction, in addition to other measures, to reduce fullness in the lateral upper lid (e.g. lateral fat pad reduction and lacrimal gland prolapse treatment).

3. The heaviness in the lateral upper lid as noted may be caused by one or more of the following:
   (a) The lateral subseptal fat pad, which can be treated by reduction similarly to other retroseptal fat.
   (b) A low-hanging, obvious orbital lobe of the lacrimal gland, which can be treated by resection or recession by sutures, depending on preference or concerns.
   (c) The ROOF, which lies over the superolateral bone and orbital septum across the upper lateral and middle lid region.

4. The ROOF can be safely reduced along the rim, although often a large vessel may require cautery. This vessel is anastomotic with the supraorbital vein medially, or if arterial with the supratrochliar.

5. Because the lacrimal nerve crosses the superolateral rim here, treatment of the ROOF may temporarily cause a small area of numbness in the lateral brow area.

6. The ROOF is part of the overall galeal fat pad, which extends upwards under the frontalis for 3 cm (±). This fat pad envelops the underside of the corrugator laterally, then continues medially to allow a corrugator gliding sleeve. It is often seen under the medial edge of the procerus muscles.

7 The galeal fat, of which the ROOF is one part, is responsible for the easy mobility of the lower 2+ cm of forehead. The mobile forehead actually exists as the muscles ride over and through the fat.

8 Because of this mobility, treatment of a droopy brow (as from facial paralysis) from above rarely works, as the glide planes are still active. Therefore, to stabilize the paralyzed brow exactly without movement or migration, the subgaleal fat needs removal so the brow can be fixed directly by anchors or another subperiosteal device.

9 Because the fat is a poor holder of sutures, elevation of the lateral brow by suturing to this fat rarely provides predictable long-term results.

10 Exposure of the ROOF, however, will provide access to the lateral corrugators where they insert into the underside of the frontalis muscles over a broad area. From here, corrugator resection medially may also proceed with ease.

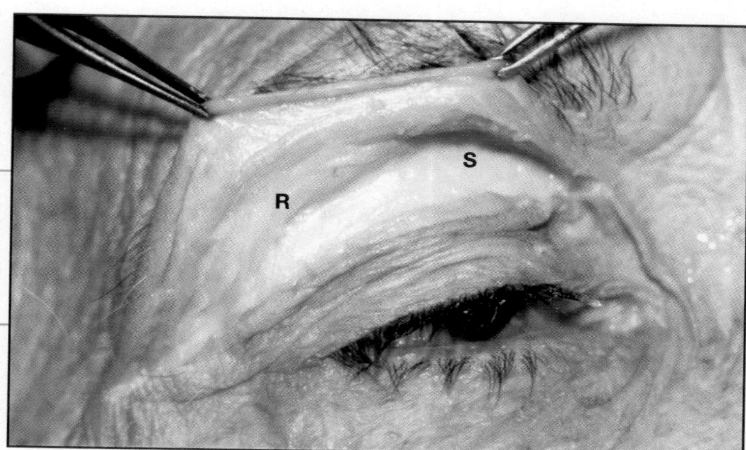

Figure 4.1

In this semifixed specimen, the orbicularis and skin are elevated to show the fatty layer, the lower ROOF (R) laying beneath it as distinct from the subseptal fat (S), as you will see.

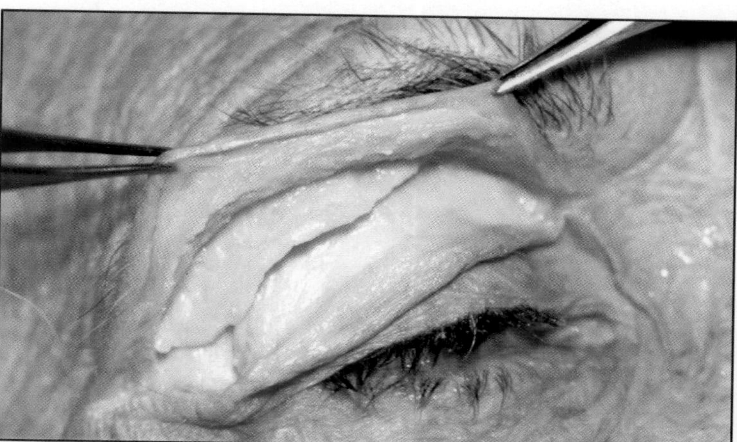

Figure 4.2

The full medial-to-lateral extent of the ROOF can be seen once the lower galeal fat pad is dissected free from the orbicularis oculi. Note how wide this can be, i.e., over the lateral rim to almost medial limbus of the eye.

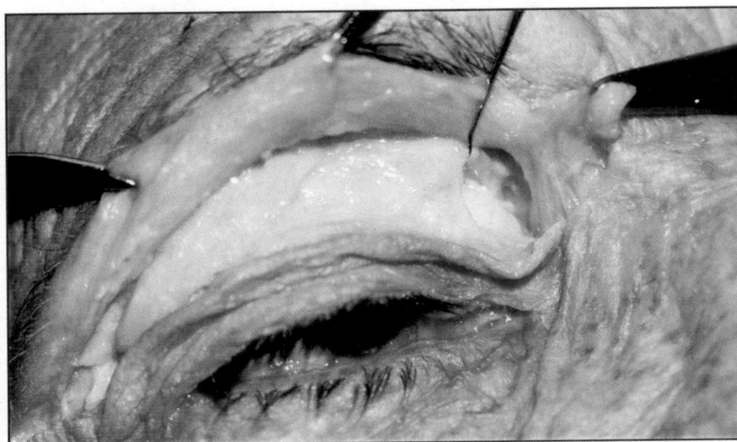

Figure 4.3A

The orbital septum is cut and the edge elevated with a hook.

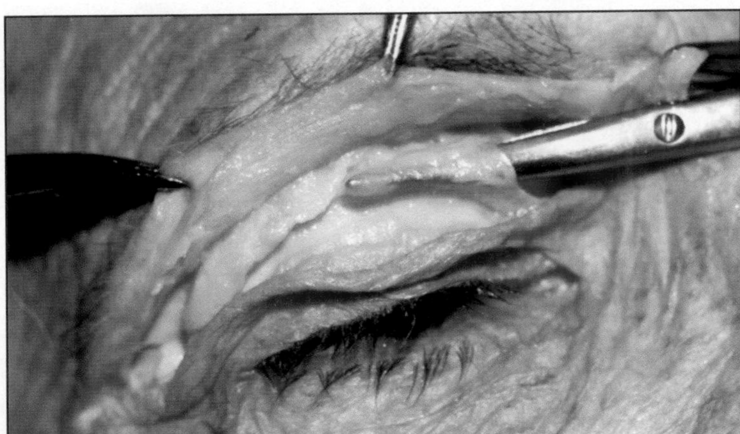

Figure 4.3B

The scissors are placed below the orbital septum from medial to lateral.

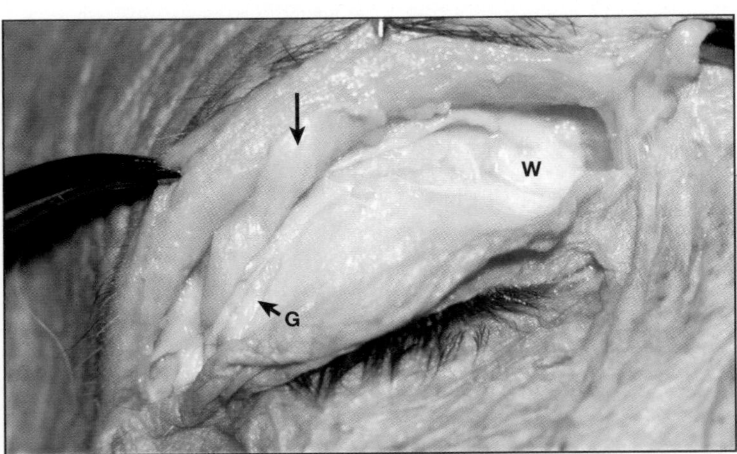

Figure 4.4

The septum is opened. White medial (nasal) fat (W) is visible, in contrast to the middle, more yellow fat. The ROOF (*arrow*) is noted as well as some lacrimal gland (G).

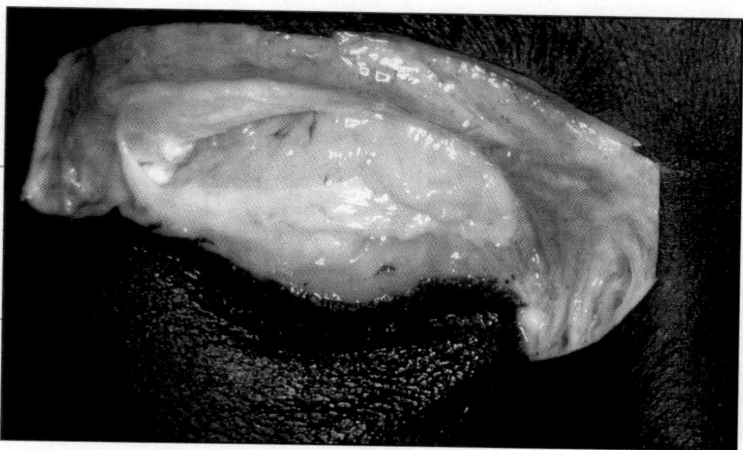

Figure 4.5A

After the orbital septum is removed in these two specimens, variations in lateral fullness—i.e., more subseptal fat versus more orbital lobe of the lacrimal gland—become obvious.

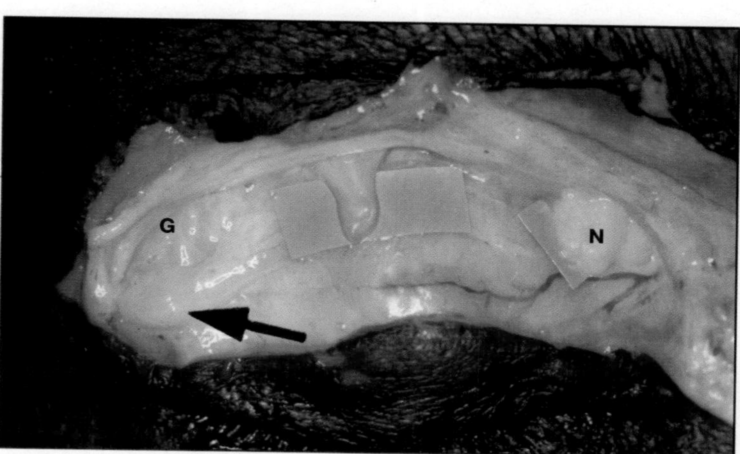

Figure 4.5B

The nasal fat is marked (N) as well as a small middle fat component. Laterally (*arrow*) there exist a large lump of fat (*arrow*) with orbital lobe of lacrimal gland (G) on top of it.

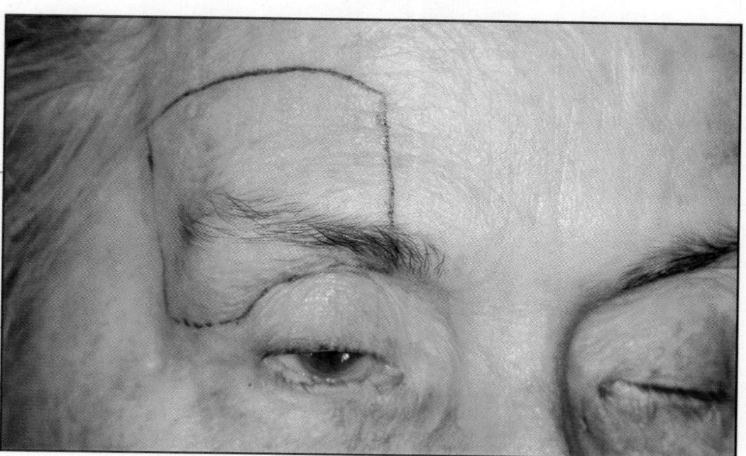

Figure 4.6

ROOF and beyond: Blue marker depicts the zone of concentration. The aim is to see the extent of the ROOF and lateral galeal fat pad, and make anatomic/surgical correlations.

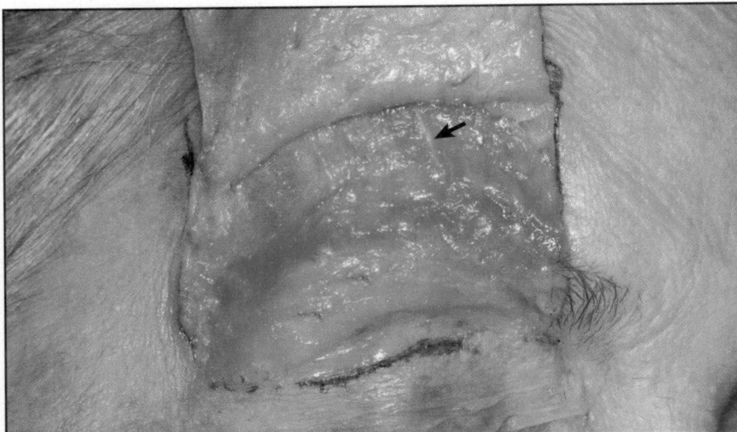

Figure 4.7

Skin alone is elevated. Note (*arrow*) sensory fibers from the supraorbital nerve travelling vertically cephalad atop the frontales muscle. The muscle is thin over the ROOF and rim.

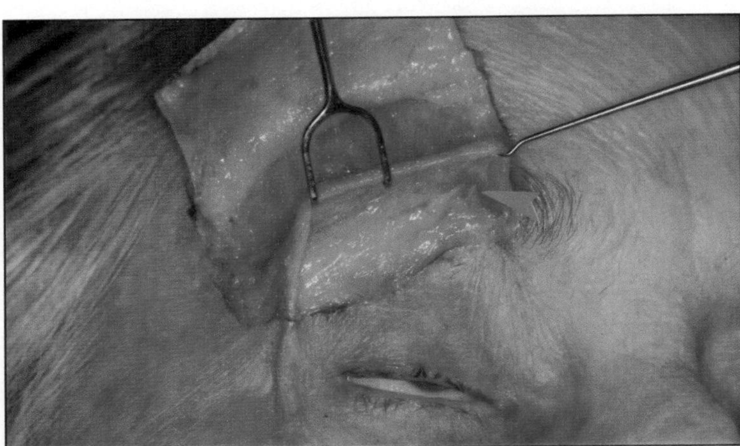

Figure 4.8

The orbicularis oculi muscle is elevated with its underlying fascia to expose the ROOF. The red dart depicts the lateral lower corrugator being exposed as it inserts into the frontalis muscle underside.

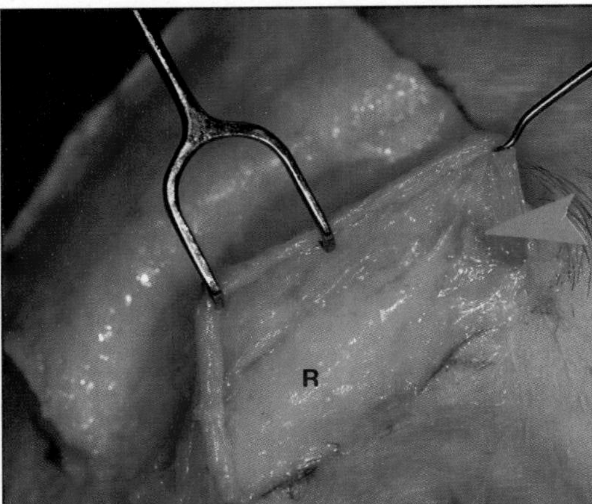

Figure 4.9

Close-up. ROOF (upper part) (R).

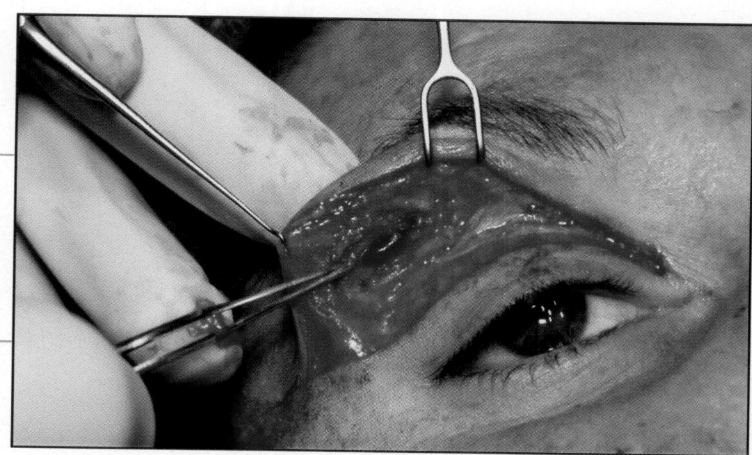

Figure 4.10

In this in vivo dissection, this vessel is quite obvious during ROOF removal, and the surgeon should be aware of it. Control is not difficult. This vein anastomosis with the supraorbital vein more medially.

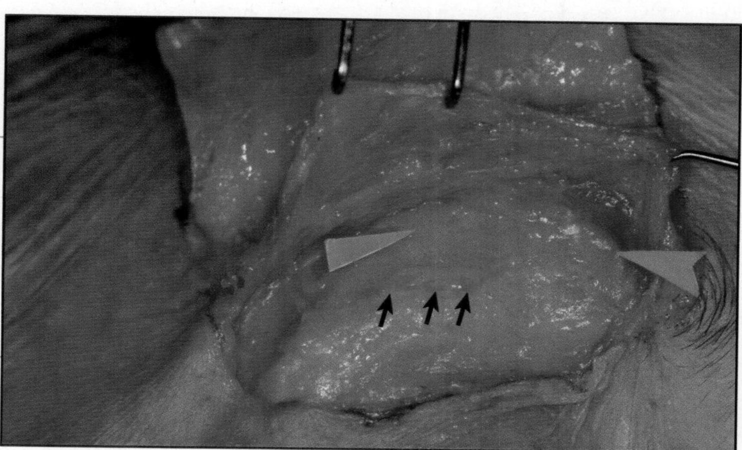

Figure 4.11

The cephalad extent of the galeal fat pad laterally is noted (*green dart*). The red dart shows the galeal fat under the corrugator, which is inserting into the underside of the frontalis muscle. The red is really a collapsed vessel from the supra-orbital region (*arrows*).

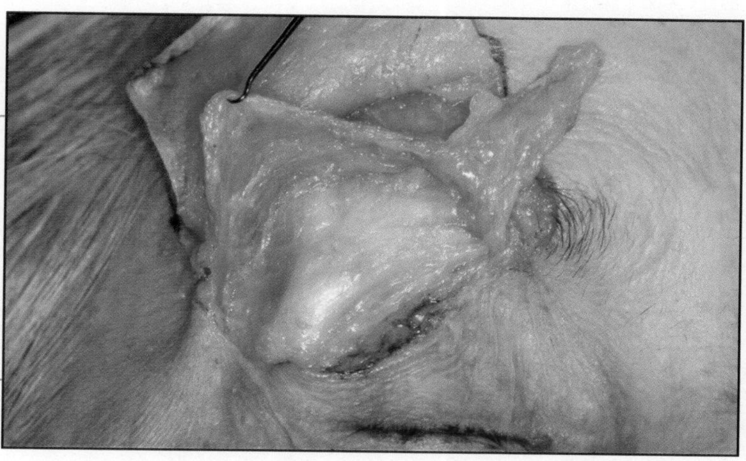

Figure 4.12

The galeal fat pad and ROOF are reflected medially exposing the bare periosteum of the superolateral rim.

Note: To stabilize the brow here, anchors or hooks may be placed in the bone with attachment to the brow. Once the fat pad is removed, the brow will stay in position.

CHAPTER 5

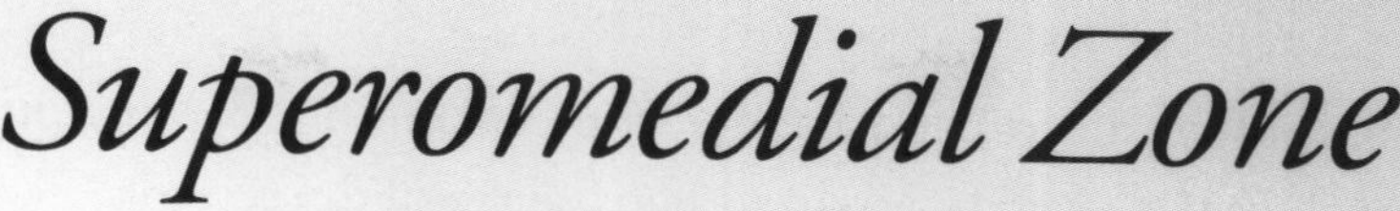

Superomedial Zone

1. The corrugators, proceri, and frontalis muscles are innervated by the frontal (temporal) branches of the facial nerve on each side. The depressor supercilii and medial orbicularis oculi are *not*; the zygomatic branch of cranial nerve VII innervates those.

2. The corrugator on one side may be of varying size, but two specific heads do not exist. The supratrochlear nerves always pass through these muscles. The nerves do not really separate the corrugator into two heads. The corrugators are panel-like muscles that require surgical diligence for full extirpation.

3. The supraorbital nerve passes under the corrugator and then through them sometimes, but usually through the frontalis to provide multiple branches vertically on the surface of the frontalis.

4. The supraorbital nerve separates into a medial (superficial) and a lateral (deeper) part, which will be presented in depth. The deep branch may exit together with the former, or separately as one to three branches, proceeding cephalad and always medial to the superior temporal line.

5. The corrugator insertion into the underside of the frontalis is 4.2 to 4.5 cm from the midline and over a large area. The origin is about 1 cm wide.

6. The muscles of the lower forehead are surrounded by fat, which accounts for their mobility in the lower forehead. This fat is all part of the galeal fat pad, which extends across the entire lower forehead on each side.

7 Distances of key nerves and arteries from the midline are presented for memorization to help in surgery, such as paramedian forehead flaps, surgical dissections, etc.

8 Vessels also course horizontally across the lower forehead; the key vessels for the supratrochlear region are *arteries*, but veins predominate about the supraorbital zone.

9 The procerus muscles are separate from one another in the midline. Under each edge, fat protrudes to assist in motion. Between the proceri in the forehead, fascia, but no muscle, runs vertically in the midline.

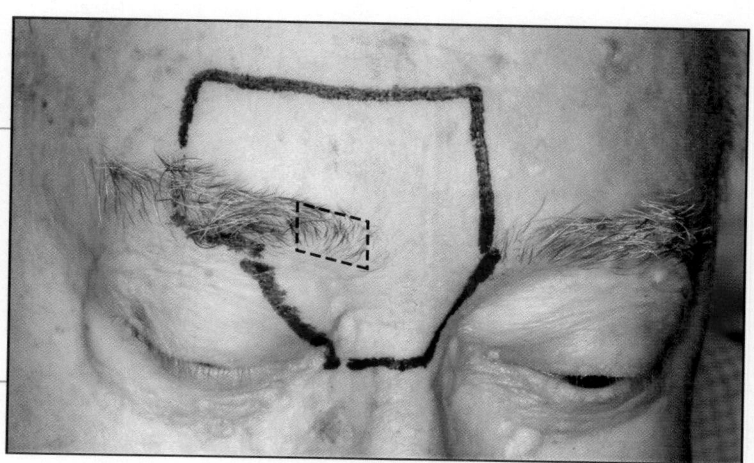

Figure 5.1

The superomedial zone. This region concentrates on the corrugators, procerus, supraorbital, and supratrochlear nerves, and some smaller muscles. Starter fact: The medial orbicularis oculi and depressor supercilii muscles have insertions under the medial brow in area noted.

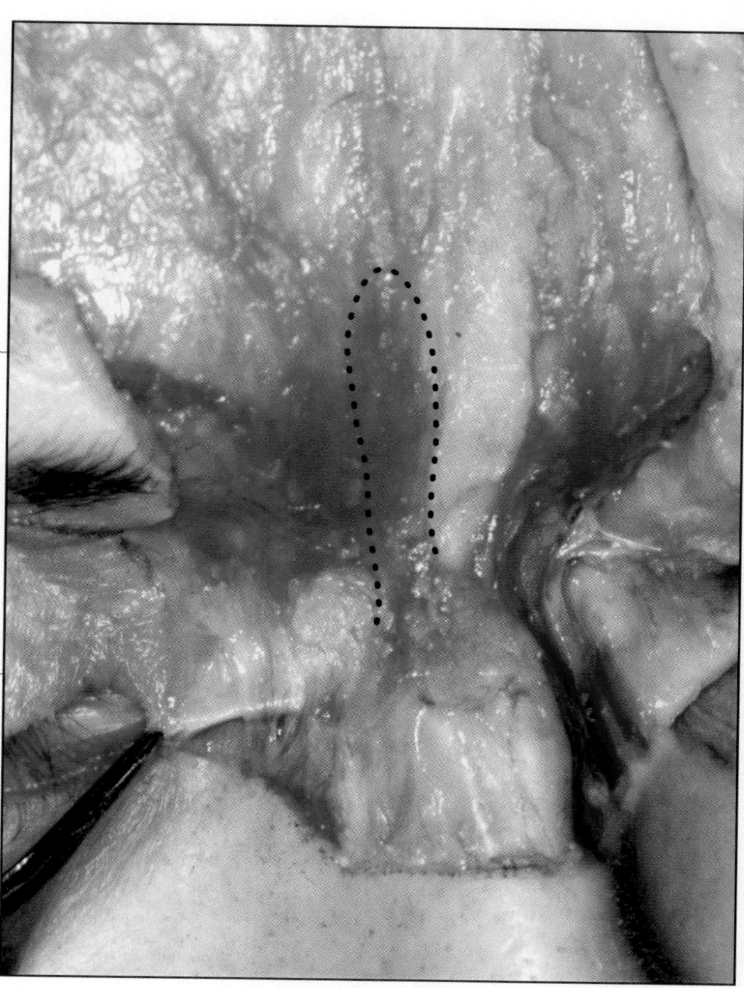

Figure 5.2

New specimen, skin off, shows the medial canthal tendon in forceps. The dotted area denotes the right procerus. Note the fascial insertion over the nasal bones in this case. Sometimes the procerus continues as muscle. The right and left always are separated in the middle. Also note that fat always can be found under the medial procerus edge, which is part of the galeal fat pad and facilitates gliding.

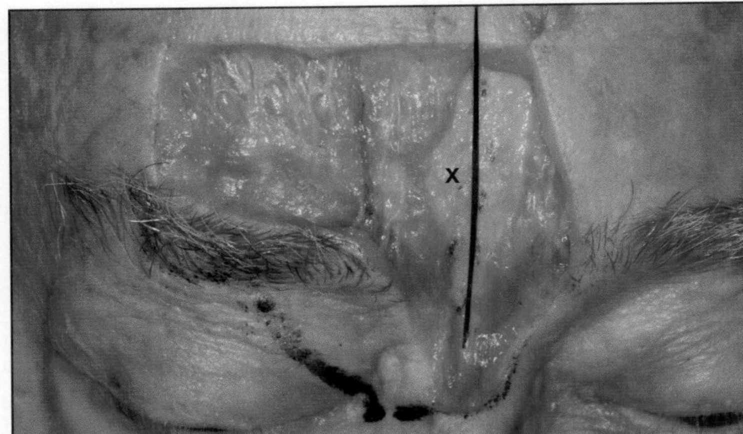

Figure 5.3

The midline is marked (*black line*). A supratrochlear vessel can be noted (*red*) to supply the paramedian forehead flaps 1.6 to 2.3 cm from the midline. Note that the fat under the medial procerus edge (X) is part of the fat glide plane.

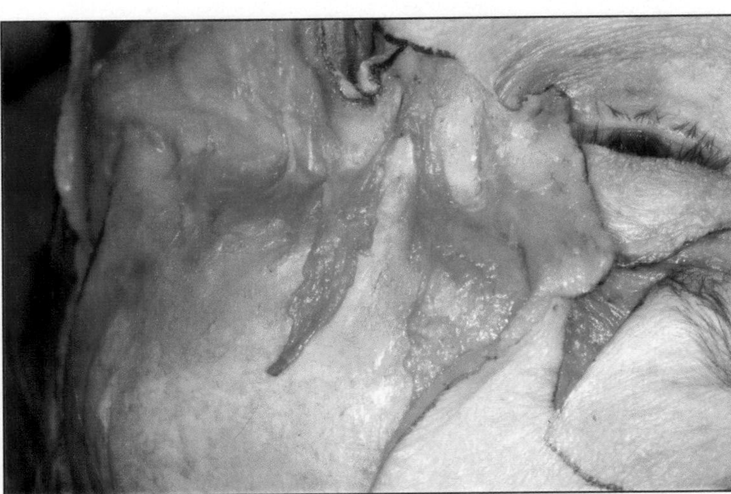

Figure 5.4

The procerus muscles are free on the left, still part of the frontalis on the right. They always tend to meet above or below the nasofrontal groove region.

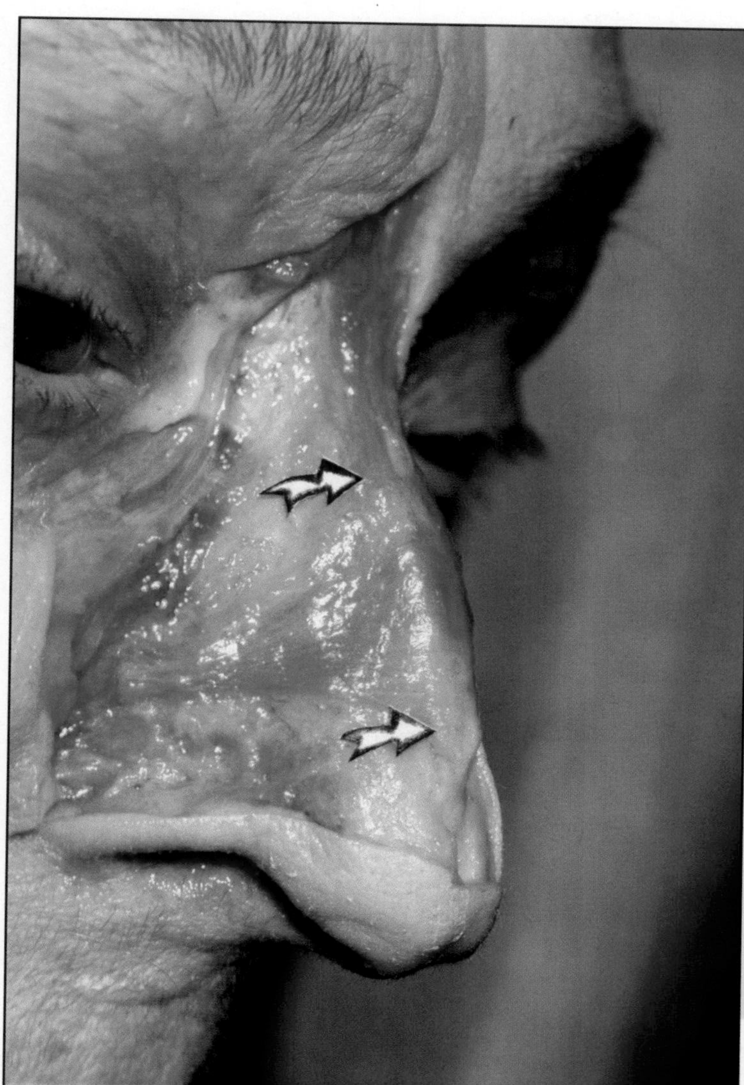

Figure 5.5

In this case, the procerus muscles proceed all the way down to meet the nasalis transverses on both sides. The arrows show the nasalis transverses insertion broadly over the mid-dorsum.

The Corrugator(s), Depressor Supercilii, and Key Nerves of the Superomedial Zone

1. The corrugator muscles vary greatly in size.
2. Distinct oblique and transverse heads (as suggested) are not present, although at times two muscles can appear separated by the nerve branches.
3. The corrugators may be quite large; therefore, residual movement, despite so-called "total removal," occurs frequently, due to partial excision.
4. The origin(s) of the corrugators on the supraorbital ridge of the frontal bone start just over 0.5 cm from the midline and cover an area of 1.0 × 2.5 cm. The vertical height may be considerable.
5. The lateral extent of the corrugators into the underside of the frontalis and beyond occurs from 4.25 to 4.5 cm from the midline. As they insert here, the muscle panels blend all the way to the lateral third of the brow.

6. The corrugators are innervated by the frontal (temporal) branch laterally, and transection or ablation of these nerves may reduce the vertical glabellar lines, but will not totally eliminate them. Nor will this prevent brow depression, as other muscles not innervated by this branch also depress the brow.
7. From the broad-based origin to the lateral third of the eyebrow, the corrugator muscle(s) courses in "panel-like" fashion in an oblique parallel direction. The medial muscle is pierced by *supratrochlear* branches, which may seem to separate the muscle(s) into separate compartments.
8. The supratrochlear nerve intrusion into the muscle varies in position. Although the supratrochlear nerves come around the rim 1.6 to 2.3 cm (average: 1.9 cm) from the midline, they penetrate the muscle with multiple small branches. The supraorbital nerve, which lies 22 to –32 mm (average: 2.6 cm) from midline, starts with a medial branch that runs posterior to the muscle bundle, and usually one branch penetrates the muscle 1 to –2 cm above the notch.
9. Endoscopic surgery to approach this muscle complex is best done with a supraperiosteal approach. The lateral corrugator muscles have fat under the insertion into the frontalis underside.
10. A large venous channel often passes from the area of the supraorbital region laterally to the fat pad retro-orbicularis oculi fat (ROOF) region. This vessel may lead to troublesome bleeding and should be anticipated.
11. Depression of the medial brow is caused by three muscles medial orbicularis, depressor supercilii, and procerus.
    a. The medial orbicularis oculi, which inserts on the medial orbital rim, has fibers that are attached to the dermis at the medial brow.
    b. Behind the medial orbicularis oculi, the depressor supercilii can be found *always*. It has one or often two small heads, with the angular artery in proximity. This muscle lies over the medial origin of the corrugator. This muscle originates about 7 mm above the medial canthal tendon and inserts into the medial brow 1.7 cm above the tendon (so it is about 1 cm long).
    c. The exact depressor supercilii origin is close to the bony medial orbital rim, slightly superior and posterior to the posterior lacrimal crest.
    d. When the corrugator muscle lies low on the rim, it may be in its oblique nature to assist in brow depression, and form oblique nasal furrows.
    e. The depressor supercilii and the medial orbicularis oculi are supplied by the zygomatic branch of the seventh cranial nerve. The procerus may be also.

    Key: Both medial orbicularis and depressor supercilii are fixed to the skin under the medial eyebrow.
12. Procerus:
    a. Courses superiorly medial to the medial head of the orbicularis oculi and depressor supercilii muscles.
    b. Arises from tendinous fibers that cover the inferior nasal bones to insert into the skin between the eyebrows. The fibers are continuous with the frontalis.
    c. The procerus muscles are connected in the midline by fascia between them and are usually separate. Under the procerus medial edge is the fat pad, which is a continuation of the fat pad that began more laterally.

Surgical thinking regarding the corrugators

1. From above, the best approach is supraperiosteal; from below, the approach involves dissection under the orbicularis oculi.
2. The vertical height of the corrugators varies greatly. The tendency is to underestimate its bulk and height.
3. The supratrochlear nerve branches penetrate the corrugator or are caudal to it, and often will be traumatized or some branches will be torn. The patient should be warned about central forehead sensory changes.
4. Adrenaline solution and loupe magnification are your greatest allies for adequate corrugator removal. Start working laterally to the supratrochlear nerves.
5. Do not forget the ancillary depressors of the medial brow, the orbicularis oculi and the depressor supercilii. And consider the procerus, which might also require transection and placement of a small filler. The procerus forms the horizontal creases at the upper radix.

Figure 5.6

Exposure of the depressor supercilii. The skin has been removed from the upper eyelid, showing the orbicularis oculi. This muscle is cut along the dotted line and flipped medially.

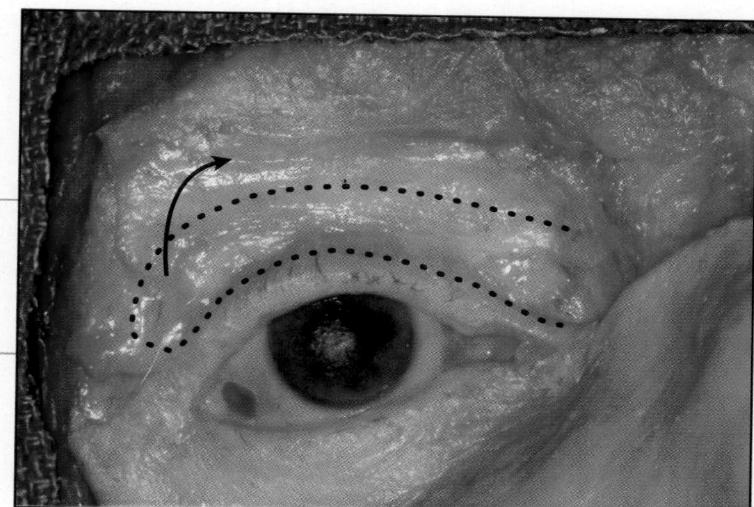

Figure 5.7

Some of the pretarsal and preseptal muscle (~ 6 mm) is elevated from lateral to medial and retracted (X). Note the reddish, vertically oriented muscle marked (*arrow*) below the medial orbicularis; that is the depressor supercilii, which originates 7 mm above the *tendon*.

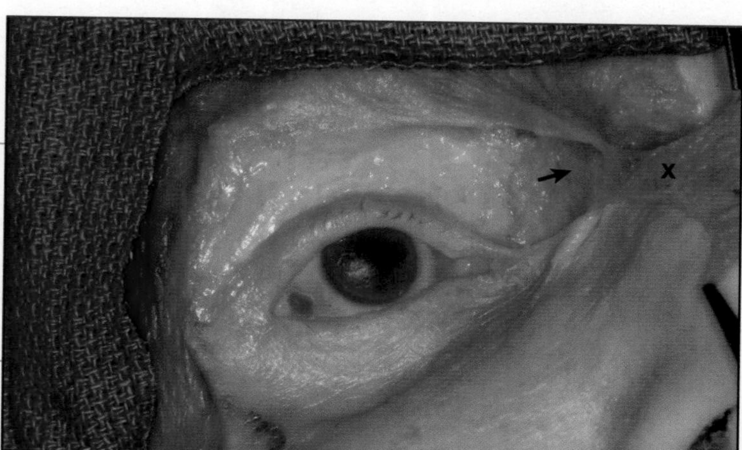

Figure 5.8

Close-up. With elevation by forceps superiorly, the red muscle (*arrow*) becomes more obvious. This muscle may possess one or two heads, and it inserts into the medial brow about 1.7 cm above the medial canthal tendon, along with some of the orbicularis.

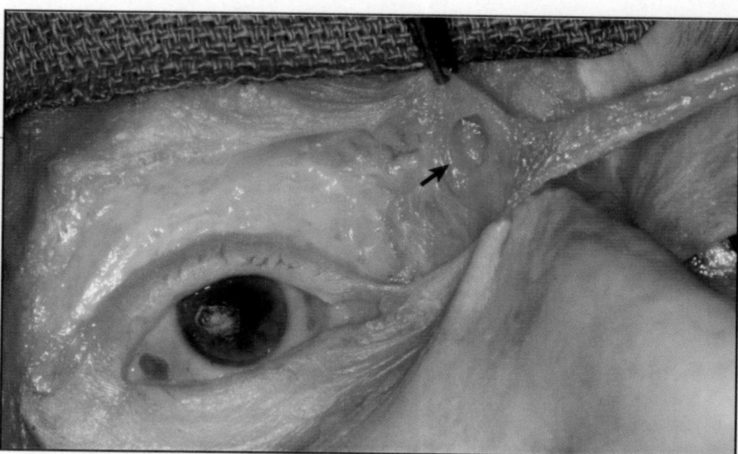

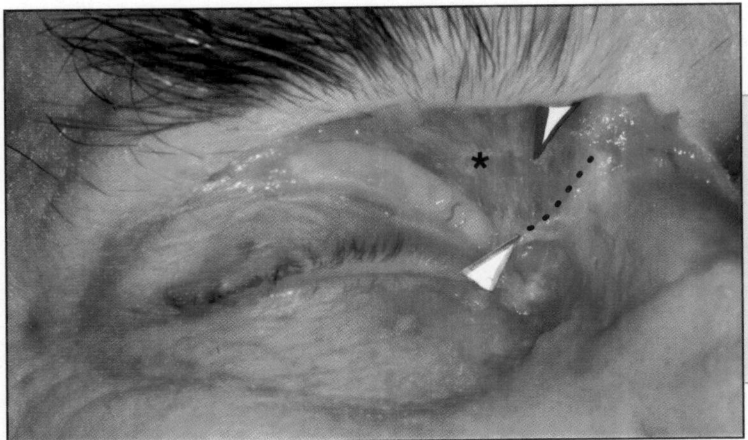

Figure 5.9

The orbicularis has been removed. The dotted edge shows where it was cut off, with the lower dart pointing to the lower edge. In this case, the depressor supercilii is double headed (see dart above and *). Between these two heads, one will find the angular artery, and behind them the corrugator. This muscle is 1-cm long and inserts into the brow skin.

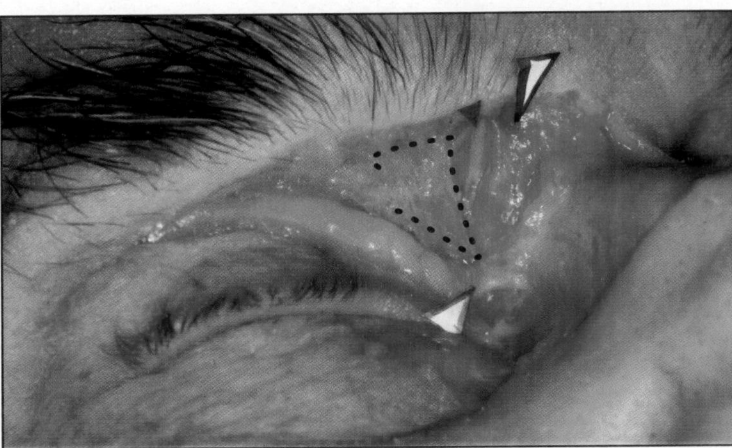

Figure 5.10

Lower dart shows the cut edge of the orbicularis. Upper dart (*blue*) shows the depressor supercilii as it is inserting under the medial brow. The angular artery is noted (*gray dart*). Note the orbital part of the medial orbicularis (*dotted*) and its connection to the medial brow. These fibers, along with the depressors, assist in brow descension. Ancillary descension would also occur with the procerus and lower corrugator, as will be seen.

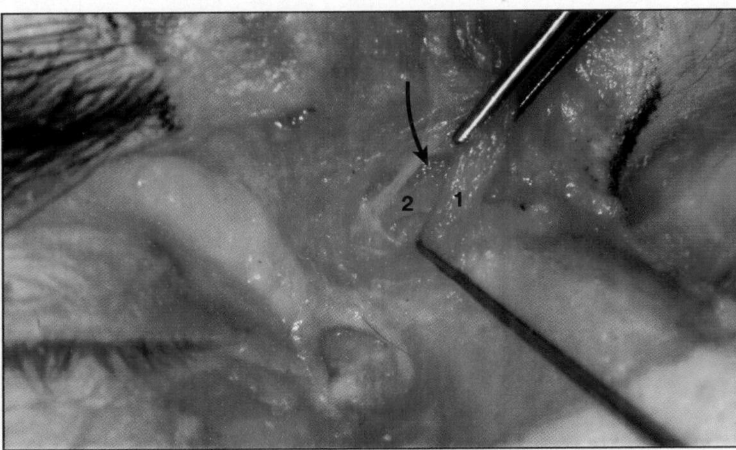

Figure 5.11

With the depressor supercilii pulled up, the medial origin of the corrugator is visible. In this case, the two heads of the depressor are noted (1, 2) with the angular artery in proximity.

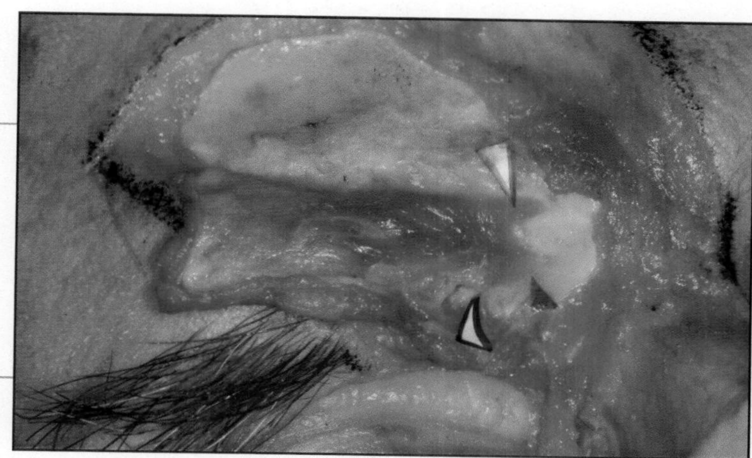

Figure 5.12

With the medial brow removed, the full extent of this corrugator is noted. Supratrochlear nerves are below it in this case. No real oblique and transverse heads are noted, unless we are to believe the upper dart and two lower darts depict rudimentary oblique and transverse heads.

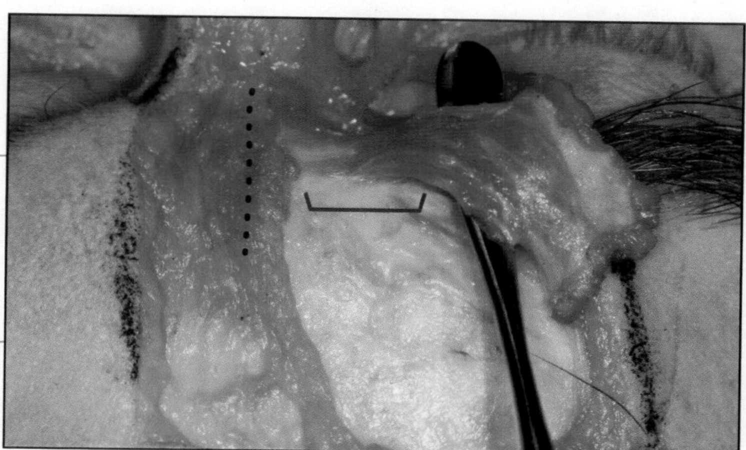

Figure 5.13

From above: More importantly, the central corrugator is lifted only to expose the 1 cm-long origin (⌴), which starts at least 0.6 cm off the midline (*dotted*). The muscle bundles appear as panels.

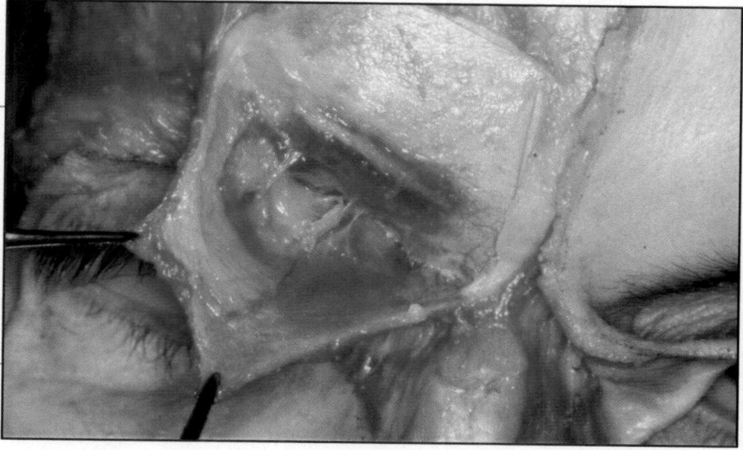

Figure 5.14

From above: The forceps are holding the frontalis forward. The corrugator is small. The supratrochlears pierce the muscle in the lower part of this narrow, unimpressive corrugator. The insertion laterally is not seen. To conceive of the corrugator as this small will leave a lot of residual muscle in many cases.

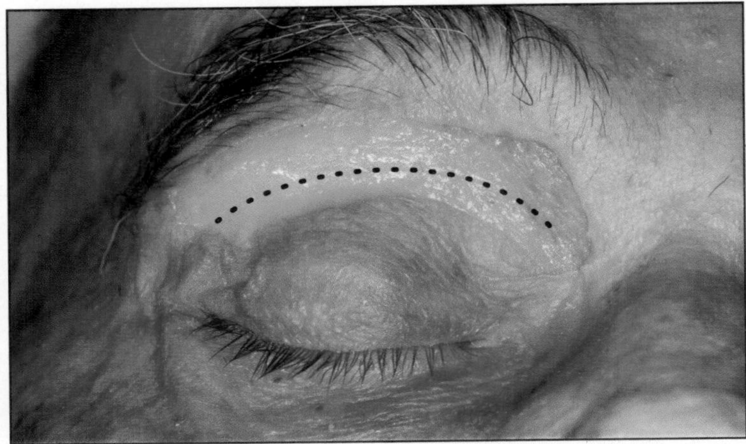

Figure 5.15

Corrugator complex no. 3: Dissecting a broader, larger corrugator complex from below. Skin is removed from the preseptal and orbital portions of the upper lid. A cut is made in the orbital part of the orbicularis oculi along the entire lid.

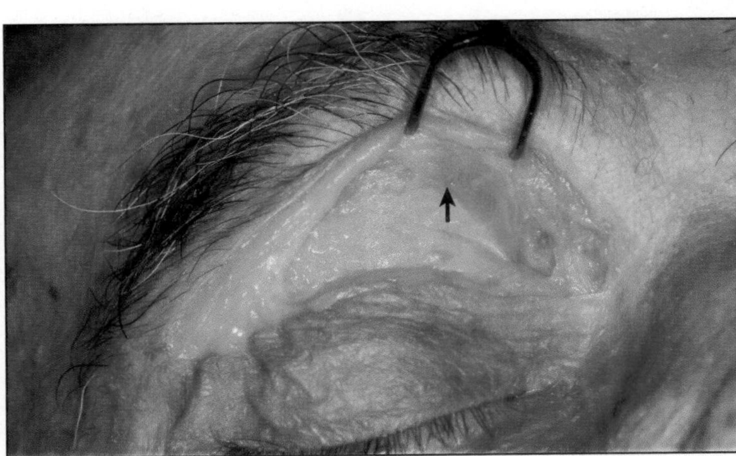

Figure 5.16

The orbicularis oculi orbital portion is held up with a double hook. Note the lateral part of the corrugator caudal part (*arrow*). This corrugator seems to be quite low and oblique.

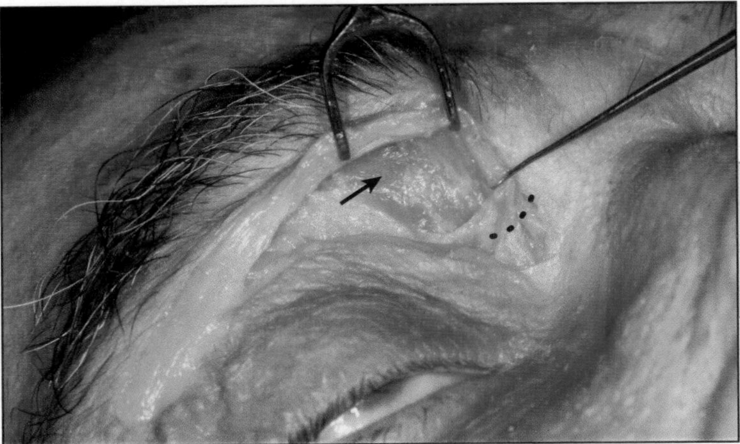

Figure 5.17

More medial elevation and retraction exposes more corrugator (*arrow*). The medial part of the orbicularis is still attached, and now it is cut along the dots.

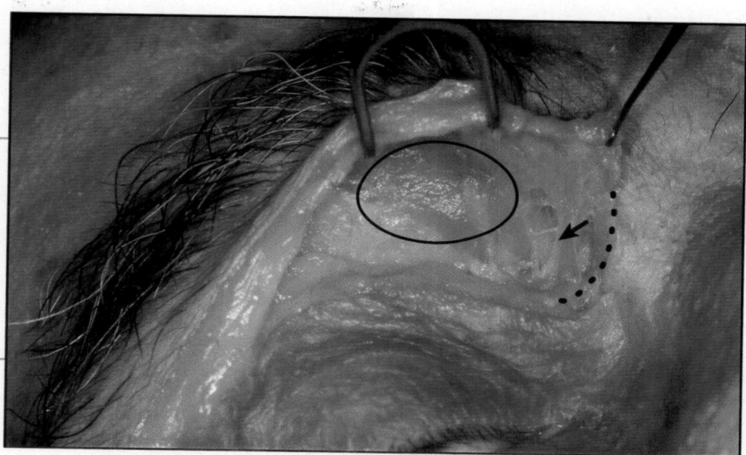

Figure 5.18

The cut edge of the orbicularis is dotted. The arrow shows a single-headed depressor supercilii that originates 0.7 cm above the medial canthal tendon to insert into the medial brow. The black circle shows an obliquely oriented lower corrugator fibers.

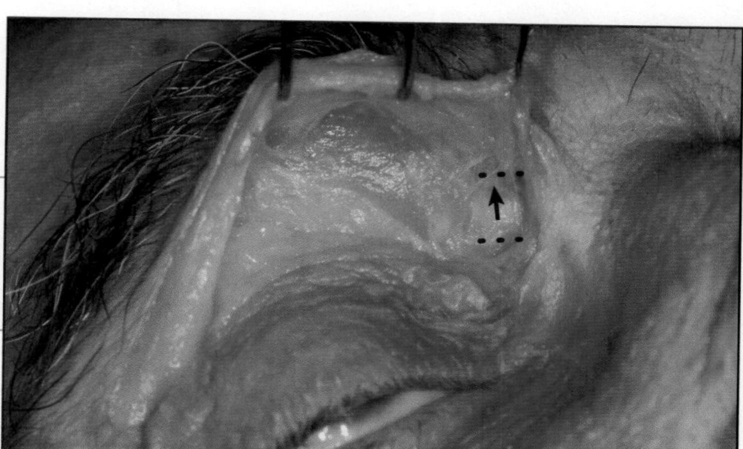

Figure 5.19

The depressor is transected (see dots on both ends). More elevation shows another corrugator "bundle" coming into view (*arrow*), and vertical nerve fibers also can be seen (see above arrow).

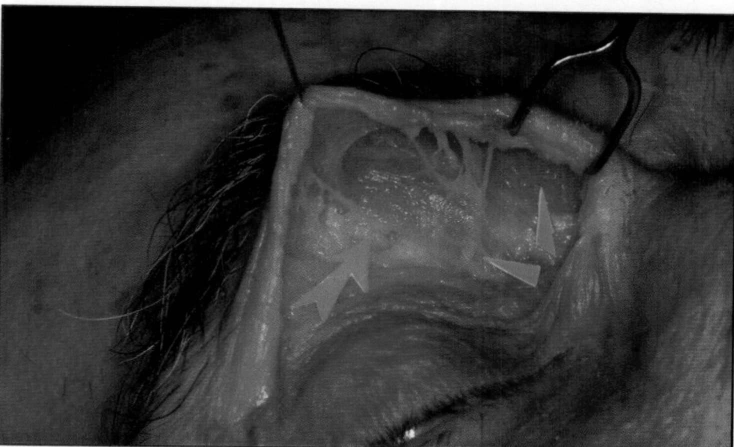

Figure 5.20

Green darts show the large origin of the corrugator muscle. Vertical supratrochlear nerve fibers are noted going toward the orbicularis frontalis junction. The red arrow shows the supraorbital nerve about 2.7 cm from the midline.

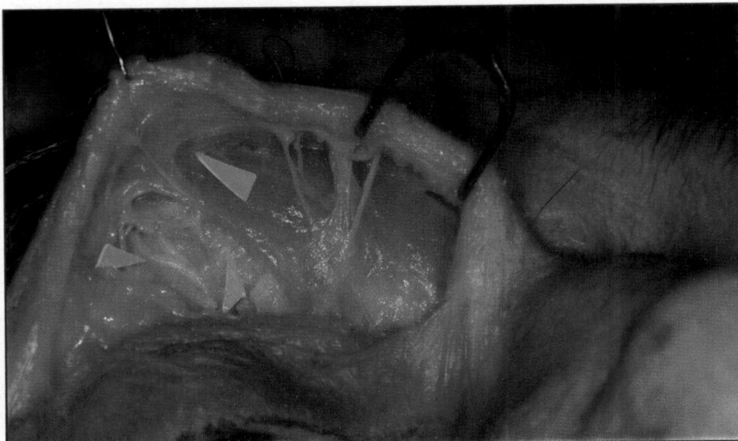

Figure 5.21

The large green dart shows the beginning of the corrugator insertion into the underside of the frontalis. The red dart depicts the medial branch of the supraorbital nerve, which may pierce the corrugators about 1 cm higher. The small green dart denotes a lateral or deep branch of the supraorbital nerve.

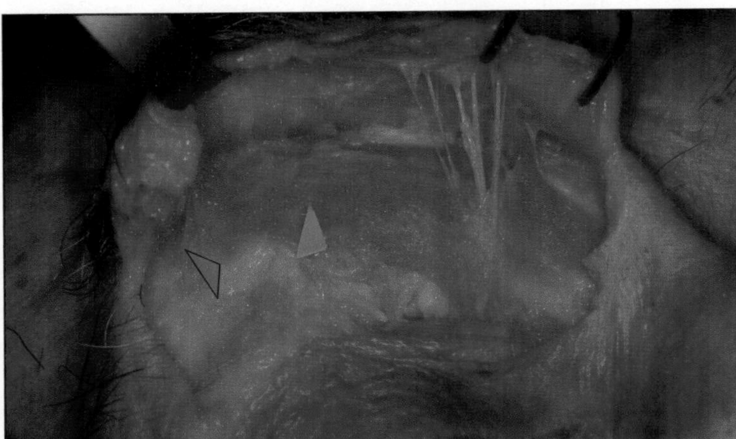

Figure 5.22

In this case, the supraorbital nerve does not pierce the corrugator muscle, despite its size, until higher up. The red and green darts show how much corrugator insertion exists on the underside of the frontalis. Thus, insertion goes at least 4.25 to 4.7 cm from the midline to the red dart.

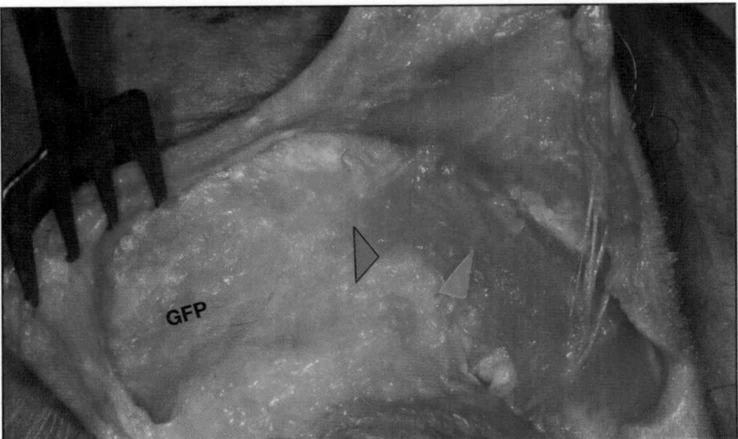

Figure 5.23

Lateral to the insertion is the galeal fat pad (GFP) or extension of the ROOF, which ends more than 3 cm above the rim. It continues medially under and around muscles to end under the medial procerus edge.

CHAPTER 6

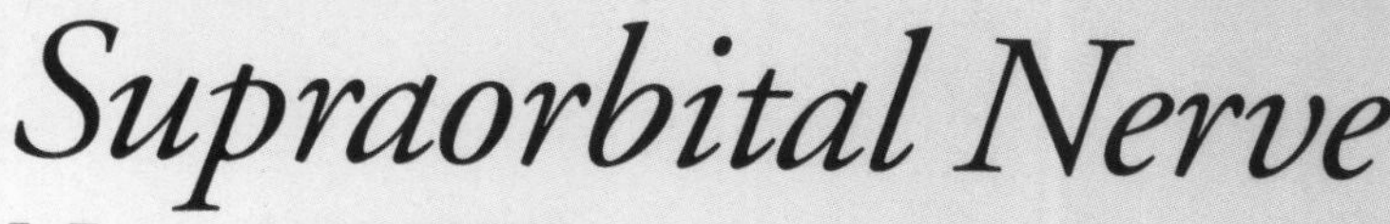

Supraorbital Nerve

Nuances/Dissections from Above

1 The supraorbital foramen/notch varies from 2.3 to 2.7 cm from the midline in men and 2.2 to 2.5 cm from the midline in women.

2 The "medial" or superficial branch of the supraorbital nerve pierces the frontalis muscle at varying levels to ascend cephalad on the surface of the frontalis muscle with many separate fibers. These nerves supply sensation to the off-midline forehead into the scalp.

3 Present always is a deep or "lateral" branch of the supraorbital nerve that runs obliquely up the forehead toward the lateral brow. This branch may exit with or from a separate foramen above or lateral to the superficial branch of the supraorbital nerve.

4 The exit foramen for this branch may be 1 cm above the rim, or along a path 3 to 4 cm lateral to the medial nerve's exit. Because the lateral or deep branch may exit above or lateral to the usual notch area, anesthetic block to the supraorbital nerve foramen region may require augmentation to anesthetize the upper lateral forehead. The needle should be passed along the periosteum above the rim from the level of the foramen and laterally for 3 to 4 cm.

5 The nerve's lateral branch usually runs between the galea and periosteum; the nerve may bifurcate or trifurcate into two or three branches as it courses cephalad. Sometimes there are small branches that may travel subperiosteally and groove the skull. These probably supply the periosteum itself. The lateral branches can always be found in the midforehead to lie 0.5 to 1.5 cm medial to the superior temporal line.

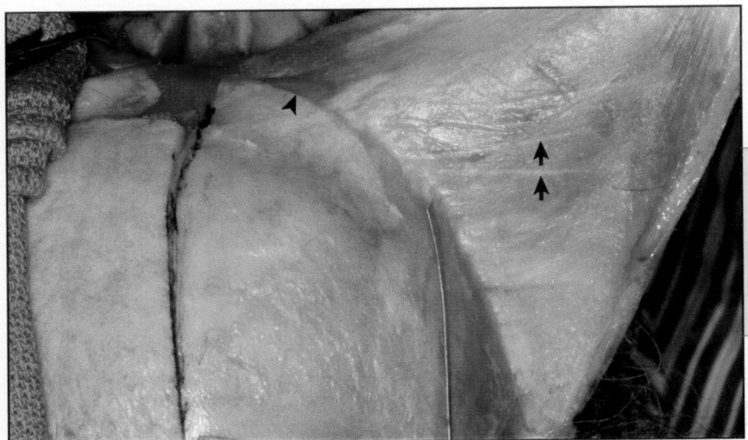

Figure 6.1

Supraorbit from above. A cut is made just to the right of the midline. A supraperiosteal dissection is done. The blue strip marks the superior temporal line. Note deep supraorbital nerve branches (*arrows*) and the corrugator origin (*dart*).

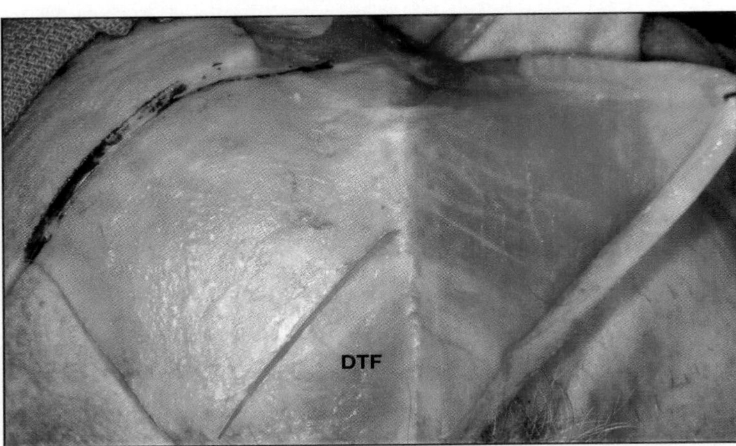

Figure 6.2

Side view. The blue strip is on the superior temporal line. The deep temporal fascia (DTF) is marked. The deep nerves would lie medial to the superior temporal line.

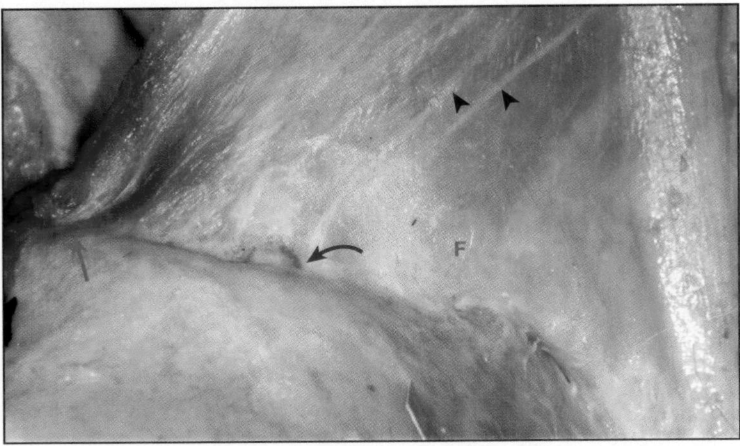

Figure 6.3

Dissection is taken almost to the rim. Note the galeal fat pad (F). There is a vessel (*arrow*) commonly seen here that goes from the supratrochlear nerve toward the retro-orbicularis oculi fat (ROOF). Deep branches of the supraorbital are noted with darts. Note the corrugator origin (*red arrow*).

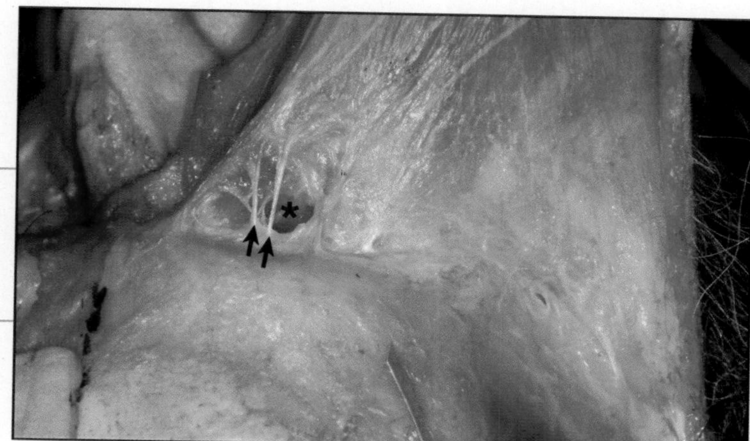

Figure 6.4

The galeal fat pad is removed from under the corrugator from medial to lateral, exposing supratrochlear nerves (*arrows*). The underside of the corrugator can be seen coming into view (*).

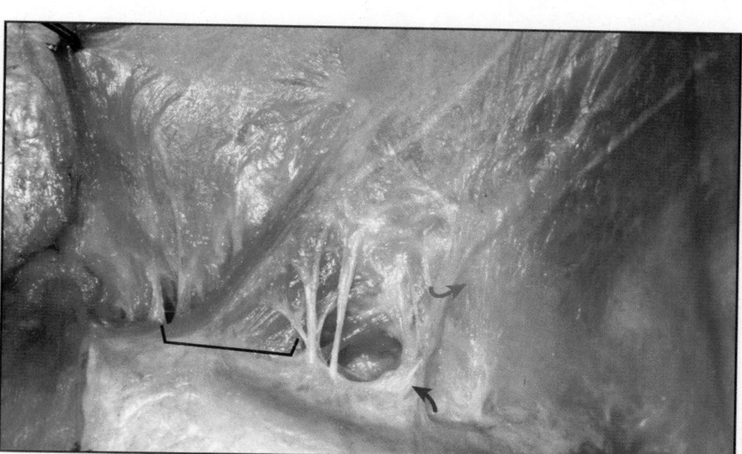

Figure 6.5

Close-up. The galeal fat pad is peeled more laterally (*red arrow*). Note the muscle bundles of the corrugator and the wide origin (⎵). The supraorbital nerve is noted (*blue arrow*), as are the more medial supratrochlears.

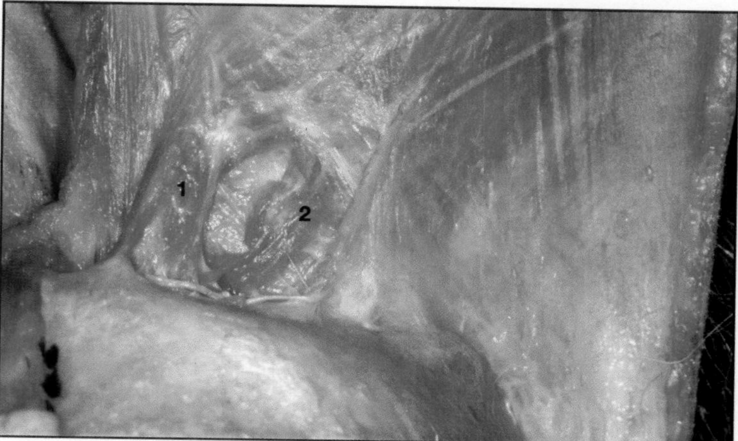

Figure 6.6

Nerves have been cut where they passed through the corrugator. Two muscle bellies (1, 2) can be artificially made, but in fact they are confluent.

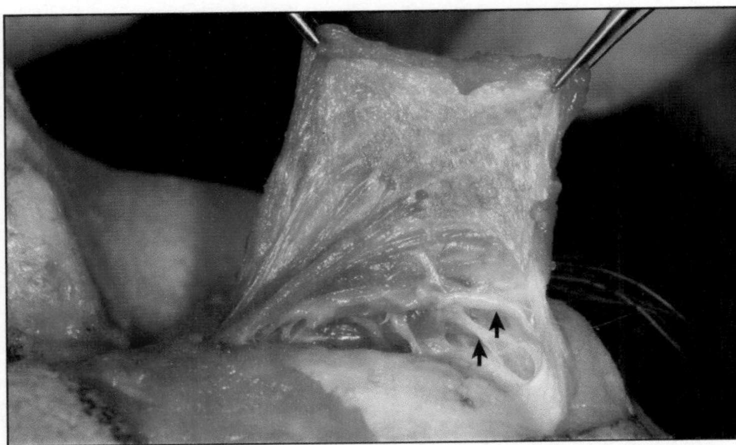

Figure 6.7

New, special dissection of the corrugators. Note the panel-like muscle configuration as the corrugators insert into underside of frontalis. Nerves (motor cranial nerve VII) are marked (*arrows*).

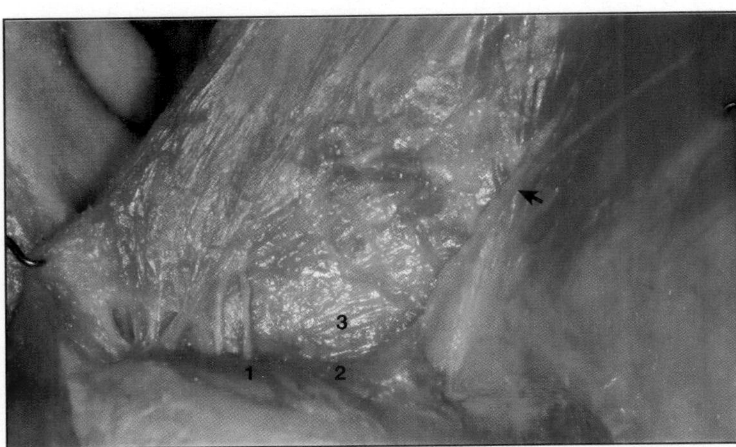

Figure 6.8

Corrugator muscles (1, 2) are flopped down. Note the underside of the orbicularis oculi (3) and the deep lateral branch of the supraorbital nerve (*arrow*). The supratrochlears (two branches) are entering the frontalis.

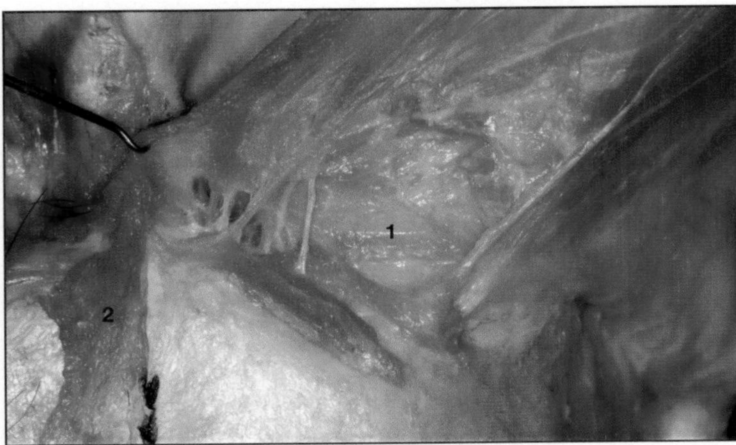

Figure 6.9

Same figure at a more anterior position looking down. Note the orbicularis oculi (1) and the procerus (2).

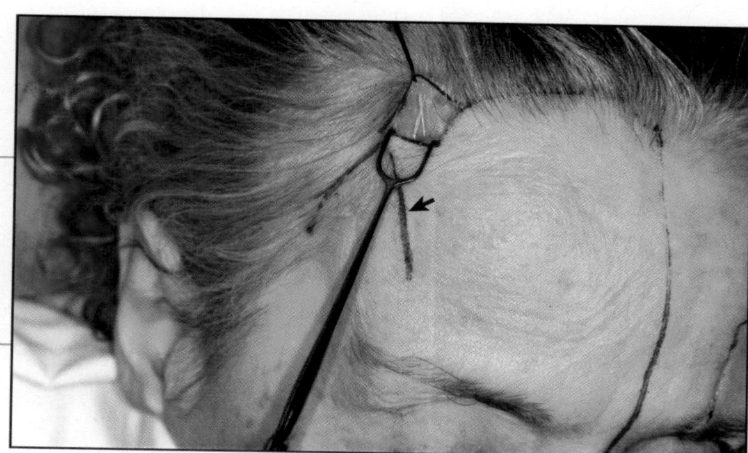

Figure 6.10

Supraorbit from above no. 2. The superior temporal line (STL) is marked (*arrow*). The deep branches are 0.5 cm and beyond medial to the STL. These branches, which are one to three in number, are usually supraperiosteal.

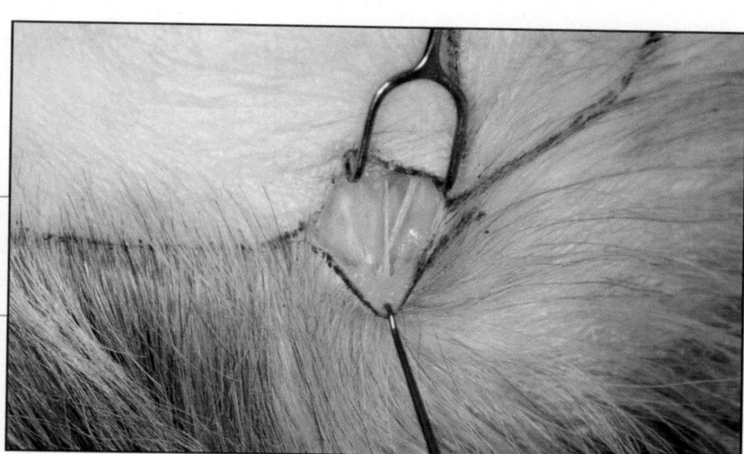

Figure 6.11

Close-up of the figure above.

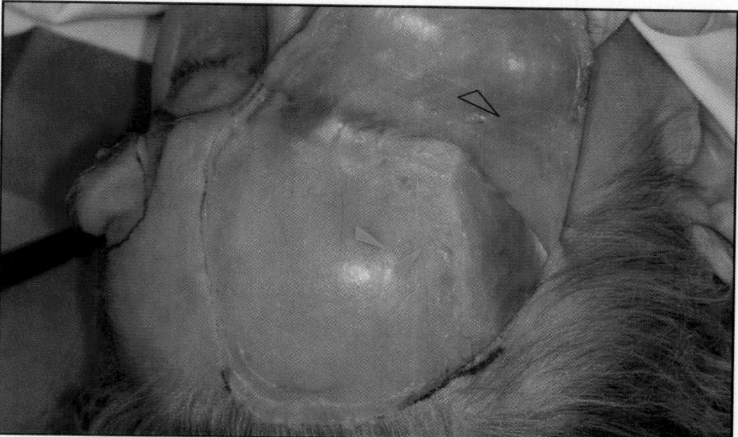

Figure 6.12

In this case, only one deep branch (*red dart*) is noted supraperiosteally. Interestingly, three nerves travel along the same path subperiosteally. Perhaps these supply the periosteum or are a variation in position.

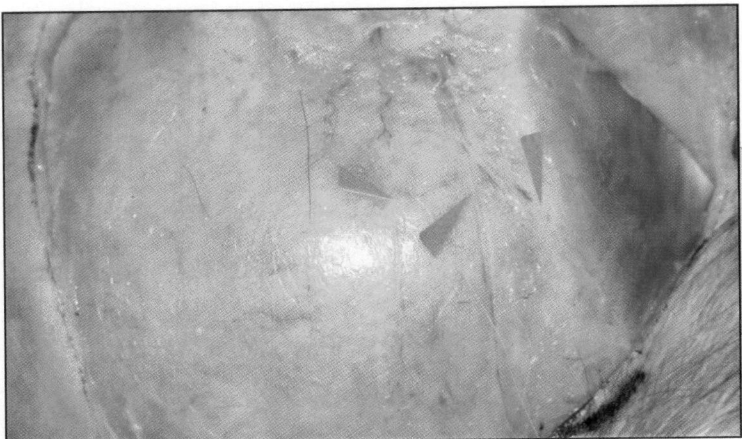

Figure 6.13

Close up: The green darts refer to the subperiosteal branches marked in the photo. Interestingly, three nerves travel along the same path subperiosteally. Perhaps these supply the periosteum or are a variation in position.

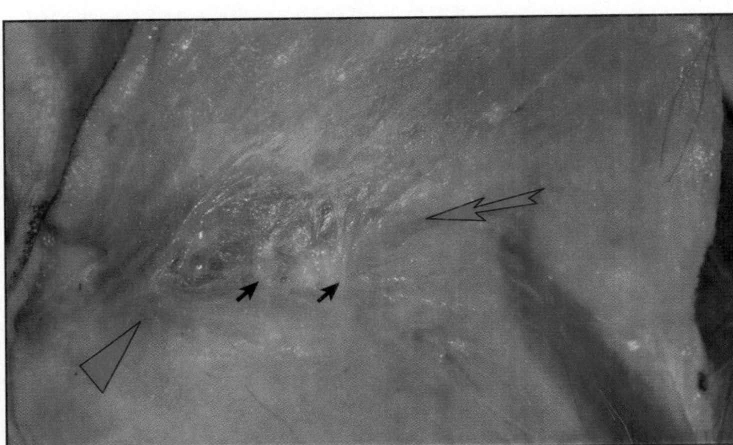

Figure 6.14

The origin of the corrugator is noted (*red dart*). The galeal fat pad (*red arrow*) is small in this specimen. The supratrochlear (*medial arrow*) and medial supraorbital (*lateral arrow*) nerves are noted.

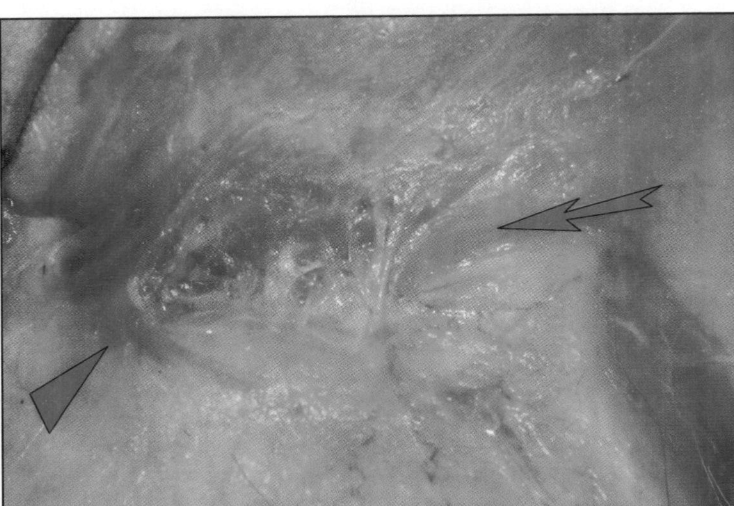

Figure 6.15

Close-up of the figure above.

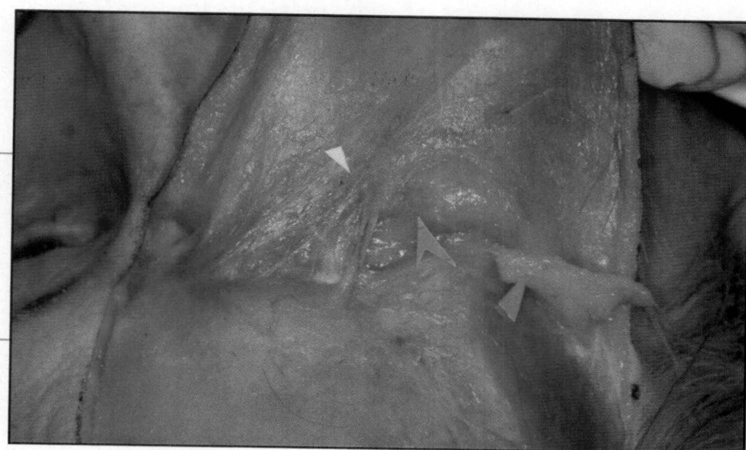

Figure 6.16

The small galeal fat pad/ROOF is removed and retracted laterally (*red dart*). The orbicularis muscle (*green dart*) is noted. The corrugator insertion into the underside of the frontalis is marked (*white dart*).

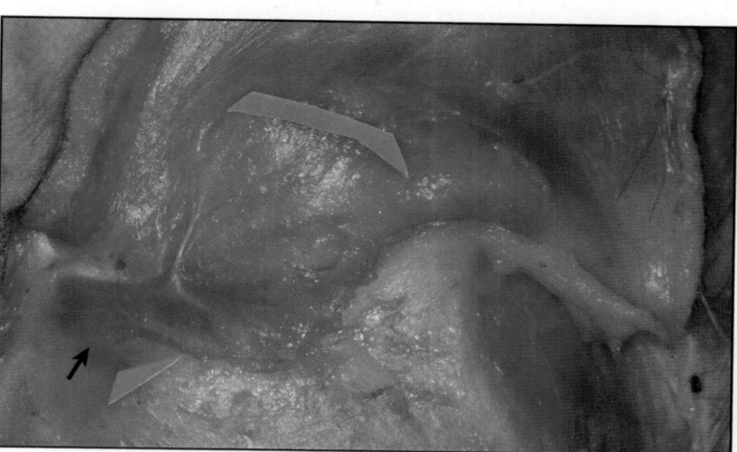

Figure 6.17

The green bracket denotes the wide area of insertion into the underside of the frontalis. The darts show this area on the muscle. There do not seem to be two heads here, just a small vertical extension at the origin (*arrow*).

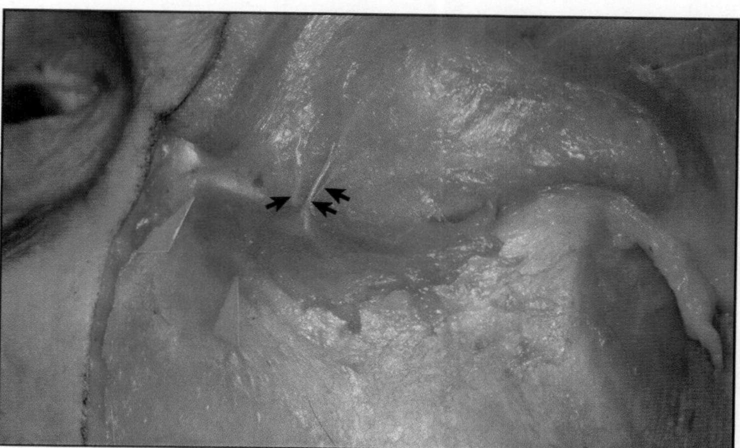

Figure 6.18

Multiple supratrochlear branches (*arrows*) pierce the lower muscle. The origin of the corrugator muscle is noted (*darts*). The muscle itself is 1.3 cm high, much smaller than in the prior dissection.

CHAPTER 7a

SPECIAL SECTION

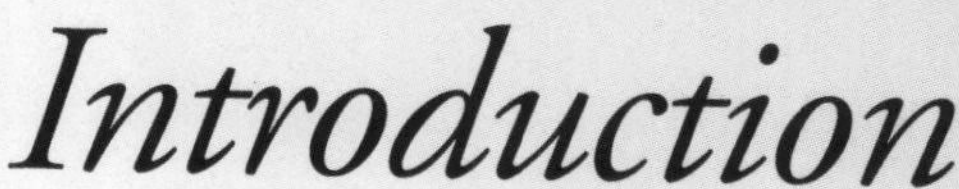

Introduction

Over the last few years, certain anatomic structures have gleaned renewed attention. They have, in my opinion, been properly discussed, and yet, the presentations of the anatomy could be clarified. Thus, each key structure will be shown in greater depth here.

7a Inferior Oblique Muscle—Its course and cautions are presented.

7b Lower Lid Retractors—The upswing in fat-sparing lower lid blepharoplasty has focused on two methods:
—Fat release via septal incision with redraping of fat over the rim.
—Fat retention via solid repair—i.e., suturing the lower lid retractors to the arcus marginalis at the orbital rim. In this mode, the fat is retained inside the rim while a "neo-septum" is made.

LOCKWOOD'S AND WHITNALL'S LIGAMENTS

7c Suspensory Ligaments—The lower Lockwood's ligament is shown again for review. However, recent anatomic findings regarding Whitnall's suspensory ligament, which depict it as a "sleeve" rather than a curtain for the levator, will increase understanding.

7d The Orbital Floor—More aggressive floor exposures for replacements with plates, nonabsorable materials, and treatment for enophthalmos justify a review of dissection parameters and the anatomic course of the infraorbital branch prior to exit from the foramen.

7e Medial Orbital Exposure—The treatment of fracture and/or exophthalmic problems, well-treated laterally or inferiorly, have not been shown clearly via the caruncle/fornix exposure, so I felt the surgeon should get a better view of this technique. Further discussion of the orbicularis oculi is included here.

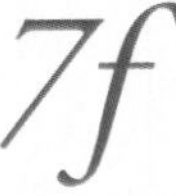

The Sphenopalatine Ganglion Block—The lateral nasal wall and its relation to the lacrimal apparatus are presented, followed by the exact method to perform this block so that the surgeon may deal with the posterior septum and turbinates more effectively.

7A: INFERIOR OBLIQUE MUSCLE (IOM)—DATA SHEET

Length:

1 The inferior oblique muscle (IOM) originates on the orbital floor lateral to the lacrimal fossa about 4 to 6 mm inside the rim. The total length is 3 to 5 cm or more, but it is best considered in thirds, with the first third starting at the floor.

2 The IOM penetrates the lower eyelid retractor complex in the middle third (for 9 to 10 mm) prior to insertion onto the lateral sclera by a small tendon, the final third.

3 Injury or even transection of the inferior oblique muscle in the first third *rarely does permanent functional damage* because the middle segment, which traverses the capsulopalpebral fascia and Lockwood's ligaments, will then act as a secondary origin.

4 As the inferior oblique muscle comes out from below the inferior rectus muscle, the oculomotor nerve innervates it. Injury here, which might also decrease blood supply just lateral to the inferior rectus, can be much more significant.

5 During transcutaneous or "distal" transconjunctival surgery for fat exposure, the large middle pocket fat should be treated first for better visualization. In addition, in the more distal approach (i.e., close to the tarsal plate) and transcutaneous approach, the first third only is usually at risk, which, as noted, has low risk for permanent sequelae.

6 If the transconjunctival (or transcutaneous) route is used, which may proceed preseptally first, then injury to the middle third is unlikely. The transconjunctival route is best done completely open to view all structures clearly.

7 With the transconjunctival *tunnel* (small incision) approach, or a more posterior retroseptal or fornix approach, the surgeon may come dangerously close to the middle or lateral final third, where nerve and muscle injury will produce serious consequences.

8 *Bottom line:* Avoid injury to the inferior oblique, especially in the middle third. Remove the central fat pad first. Stay preseptal when possible.

Figure 7A.1

The inferior oblique is marked (*arrow*) after fat removal. The first third is visible as it enters the capsulopalpebral fascia (*). Blue dots denote the lower lid retractors as they continue upward to insert "tarsally." The lower lid retractors can be sutured to the arcus marginalis to retract the fat. The inferior oblique muscle arises from a small depression or roughness on the orbital plate of the maxilla, just behind the margin and slightly lateral to the nasolacrimal fossa. The only extrinsic muscle to originate from the front of the orbit then courses posterolaterally on a path similar to that of the superior oblique tendon. The upper aspect of the muscle is first in contact with fat. It then courses inferior to the inferior rectus, prior to spreading out and inserting onto the posterior temporal aspect of the globe.

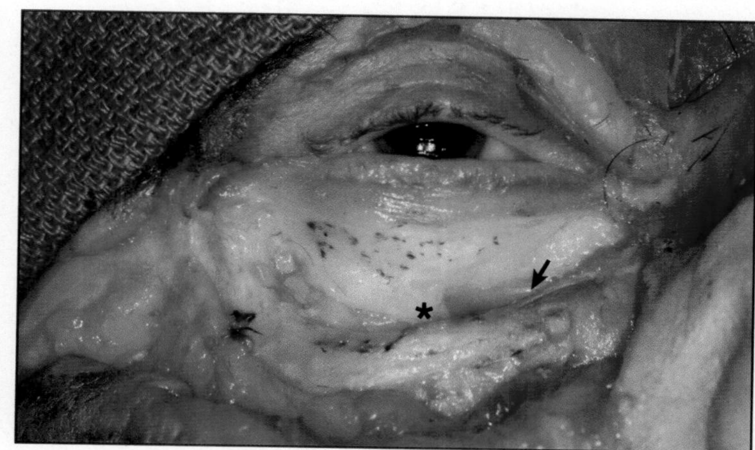

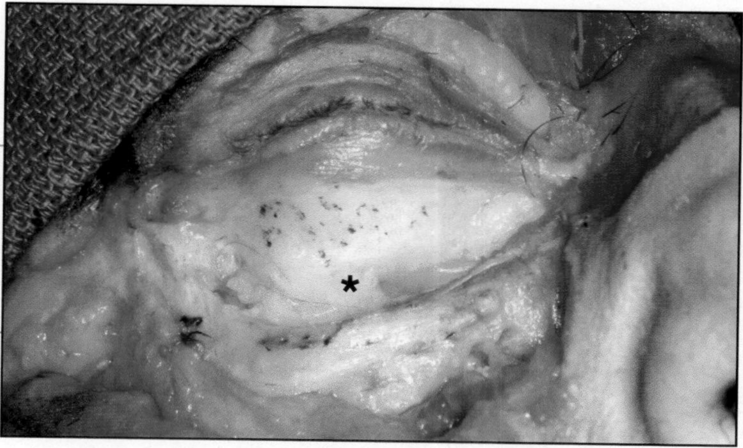

Figure 7A.2

Pulling up the lower lid shows the middle third of the inferior oblique muscle entering the fascia/Lockwood's ligament complex (*). The width of the lid retractors is at least 80% of the lid.

CHAPTER 76

Lower Lid Retractors

1 The lower lid retractors are fascial extensions (the capsulopalpebral fascia) off the inferior rectus muscle, which inserts into the lower tarsal plate, an analog of the levator in the lower lid.

2 When a person looks downward (using the inferior rectus), this extension also pulls the lid down a bit so it does not get in the way of looking downward.

3 Therefore, in lower lid reconstructions where the retractors are lost and, e.g., cartilage replaces the lower lid fascia, the lid will not move down with down gaze, so walking down stairs or reading may be problematic and require adjustment.

4 There exists, however, some substance and laxity to these retractors, so sutures will hold well. In addition, after lid retractor transection via the transconjunctival incision, separate reapproximation is unnecessary.

5 Recent efforts at cosmetic lower lid blepharoplasty have aimed at nonremoval of fat or repositioning of fat over the rim to correct tear-through problems or deficiency there. Others have suggested keeping the fat by pushing it back inside the orbit.

Suturing the orbital septum is problematic because its thinness varies, and the older patient may have an evanescent orbital septum. To keep the orbital volume and replace the fat, suturing the lower lid retractors where they are close to the rim has worked well. Running simple sutures from a lower lid retractor to the arcus marginalis (the junction of the periosteum and periorbita) works very well and will hold up long term.

Although, in theory, this procedure would seem to reduce lower lid motion on down gaze, this complaint does not arise.

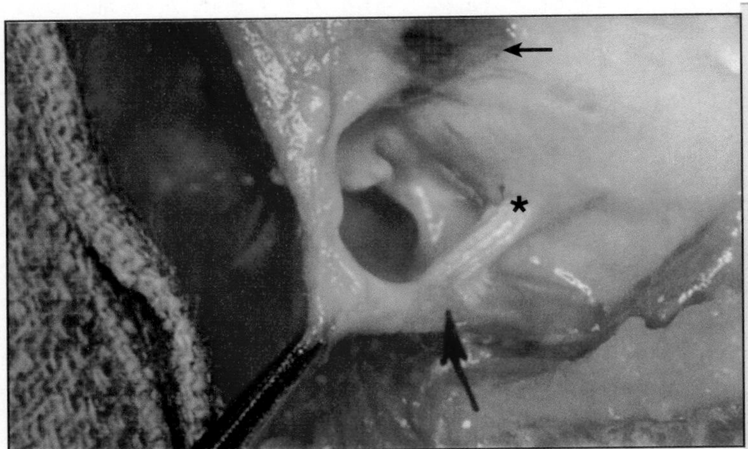

Figure 7B.1

A piece of blue rubber has been placed in the inferior cul-de-sac (*upper arrow*). The orbital septum has been completely removed. The lower forceps grasp the capsulopalpebral head just as it comes off the inferior rectus muscle (*arrow*). This capsulopalpebral fascia, known as the lower lid retractor system, inserts into the lower tarsus and conjunctival fornix. The tendinous insertion of the inferior rectus onto the globe can be seen (*). Also arising from this capsulopalpebral fascia (or lower lid retractor) is the nonstriated inferior palpebral muscle, a counterpart to Müller's muscle in the upper lids.

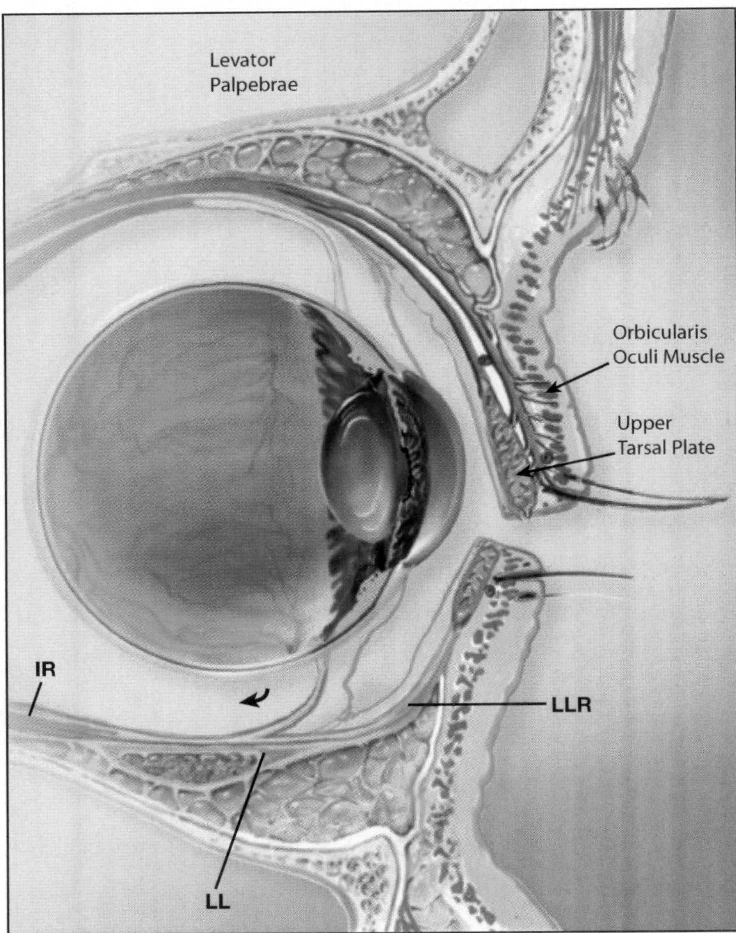

Figure 7B.2

One can see that if the inferior rectus (IR) were to move back, the lower lid retractors would pull down the lid. The green is a cross-section of Lockwood's ligament (LL), as will be seen.

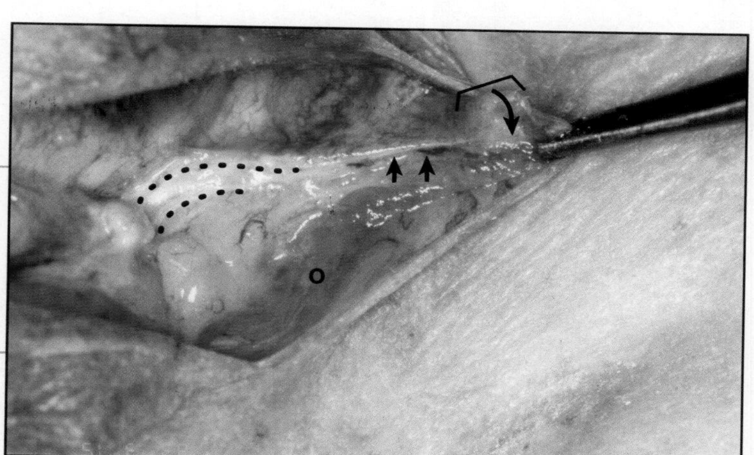

Figure 7B.3

The midlid is cut to bone. Note the tarsal plate (⌐), the orbicularis oculi (O), the distal lower lid retractors (↑↑), and the thicker fibro-fatty complex from the more proximal part of the retractors (*between the dots*).

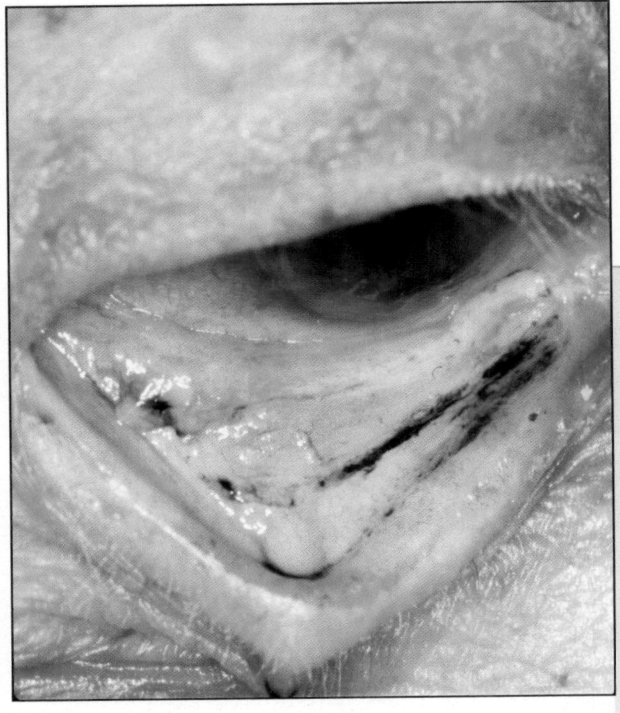

A

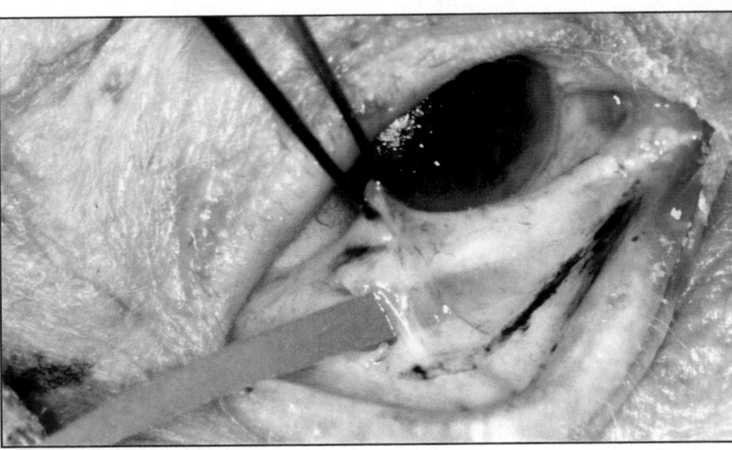

B

Figure 7B.4A–B

For fat removal or orbital floor exploration, the best transconjunctival approach is full lid, a few millimeters below the inferior tarsal plate. This incision then exposes the lid retractors (over the red tape in 4-B). *In vivo,* a scissors is opened under the retractors, and the retractors are cut from lateral to medial in one cut. There really is no reason to make small holes. The surgeon may leave this open for rapid healing or place one or two sutures to prevent prolapse of tissue. Also partial closure may prevent ointment from getting into the incision.

Following full transection of lower lid retractors, applicator buds (cotton swabs) are used to push the muscle off and approach preseptally. This is the safest method, and the surgeon should deal with the middle fat first.

A fornix incision is more troublesome for a couple of reasons. First, it puts the surgeon right into the fat without a way to gauge what to remove. Second, especially in a patient with a hypoplastic maxilla, the inferior oblique muscle is at higher risk.

CHAPTER 7c

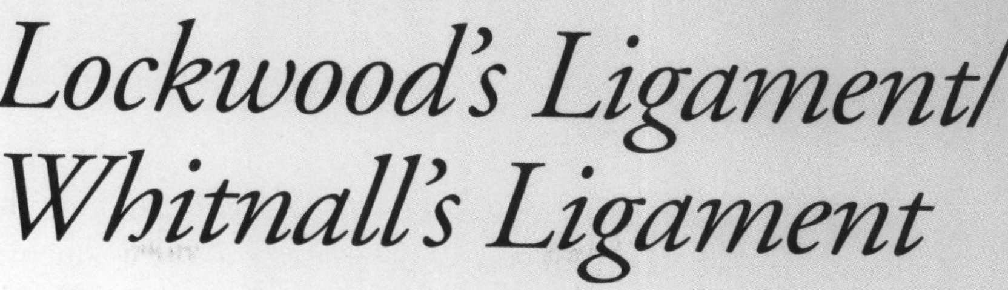

Lockwood's Ligament/ Whitnall's Ligament

LOCKWOOD'S LIGAMENT

1. The lower lid tarsus is 3.5 to 4 mm. Lockwood's ligament is about 20 mm back from the inferior tarsal border.

2. Lockwood's ligament helps prevent descension of the globe with loss of other inferior bony support. Think of it as a hammock.

3. If this ligament is caught in a blowout fracture, hypoglobus (lowered globe) will result.

4. The inferior rectus and inferior oblique muscles are intimate with this structure. Some strabismus surgery naturally may separate these muscles from their fascial associations with this ligament.

WHITNALL'S LIGAMENT

1. The upper lid tarsal plate is 9 to 11 mm, and Whitnall's ligament is 25 mm above that. The levator aponeurosis travels for 30 mm from the tarsal plate, and the levator muscle starts at 40 to 45 mm from the tarsus.

2. In cases of severe congenital ptosis, some surgeons will cut this ligament as part of a large levator resection to allow the levator muscle to come forward.

3. Whitnall's ligament actually has a superior component and an inferior component. The superior component, visible on the levator surface, is attached medially to fascia around the trochlea of the superior oblique. Laterally, the ligament splits the lacrimal gland (it helps support the gland and is adherent to its stroma) and attaches to the orbital wall laterally.

4 Whitnall's ligament in some cases may be a taut band; in other cases, a flimsy one. The taut ligaments can help repair the severe ptosis cases, as the ligament may assist in eyelid suspension as opposed to the frontalis sling.

5 The less well-known inferior component, also a fibrous band, may be found on the underside of the levator running horizontally to join the medial and lateral extensions of the superior component.

6 Thus, the superior and inferior components of Whitnall's form a sleeve of fibrous connective tissue surrounding the levator. It is not just a thickening of fascia on the top surface.

7 This mobile sleeve thus supplies support to the upper lid, acting as a fulcrum during upper eyelid motion.

8 This inferior component may convert the A-P vector of the levator to a more vertical one during upper lid movement. It is visible as a yellowish-white band over the superior edge of Müller's muscle.

9 The inferior component is continuous with the fascial sheath of the superior rectus centrally. In the region of the fornix, it contributes to the suspensory ligament of the superior fornix.

10 The medial peritrochlear attachment of the Whitnall's ligament sleeve is stronger than the lateral.

Figure 7C.1

The inferior oblique muscle (supplied by the inferior division of the oculomotor nerve) is noted (*). The muscle penetrates the bulbar fascia just as it nears the inferior rectus. The lower portion of this fascia is condensed to form a hammock-type ligament that supports the globe. The anterior portion of this suspensory ligament of Lockwood can be appreciated (*arrows*). This structure may prevent ocular descent after partial maxillectomy. Lockwood's ligament attaches laterally and forms part of the lateral retinaculum. The medial attachment seems less distinct.

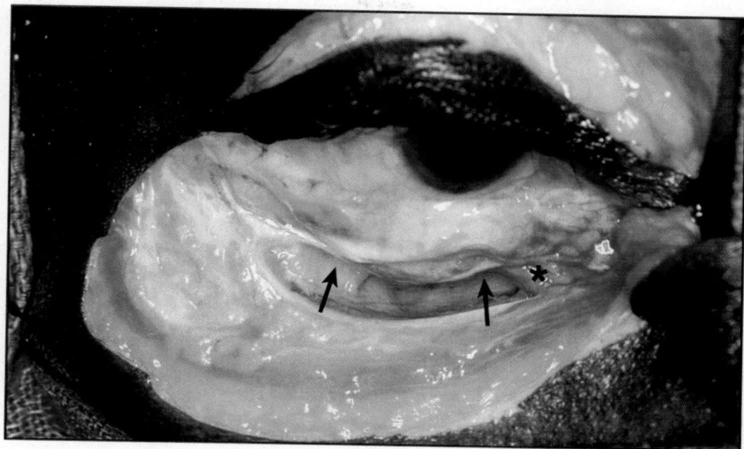

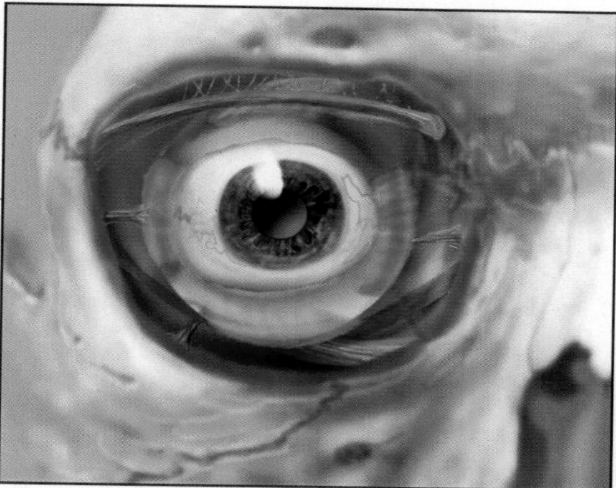

Figure 7C.2

Whitnall's ligament upper sleeve part only (*green*) appears above, and Lockwood's ligament (*green*) appears below the orbit.

Figure 7C.3A–D

Whitnall's ligament varies in size and thickness. In **A** and **B**, the superior component is thin (*red arrows*). It seems thicker in 7C–C and D. It is 25 mm above the tarsal plate (*dotted*), which is visible after the levator aponeurosis was removed and rolled up. Do not forget there is an inferior component to Whitnall's, which means that the levator actually has a sleeve around it. (In **A**, X indicates the superior oblique tendon.) The black line denotes the trochlea.

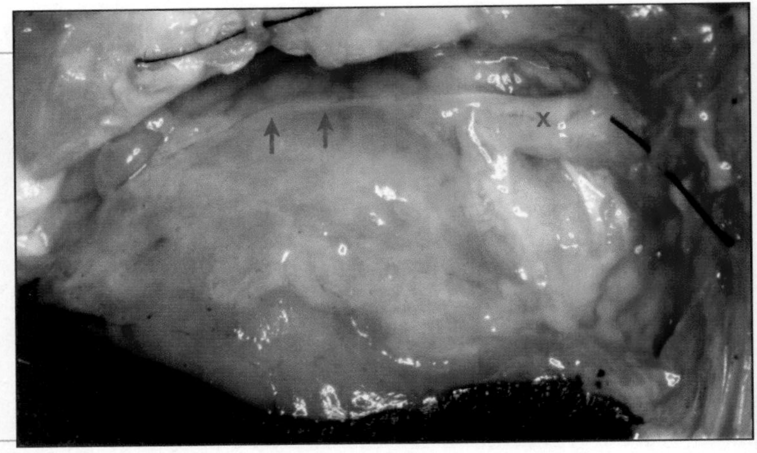

A

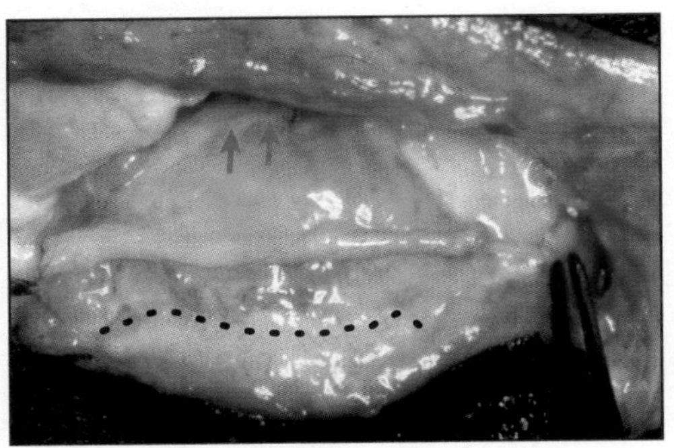

B

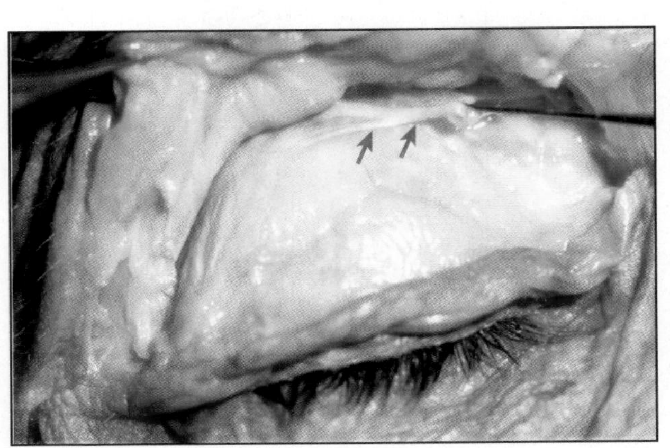

C

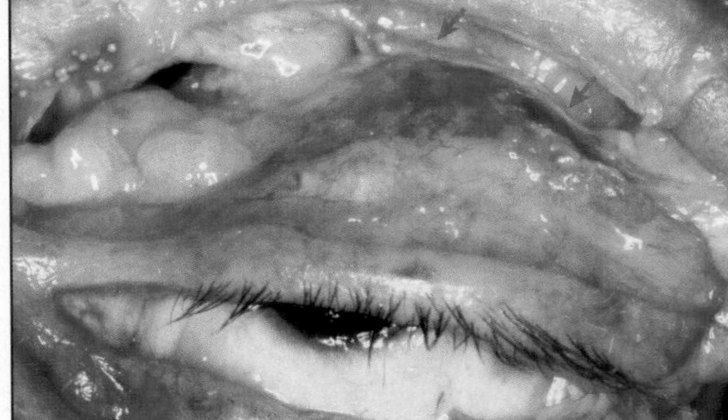

D

CHAPTER 7d

Some Thoughts on the Orbicularis Oculi

HOW TO APPROACH THE MEDIAL ORBITAL WALL FOR FRACTURE OR DECOMPRESSION

1 The lower orbicularis oculi muscle is attached to the orbital rim medially (~50%), and laterally to the suborbicularis oculi fat (SOOF) and rim by orbital retaining ligaments. Thus, ligamentous release and transection of the muscle along the rim will allow the skin, muscle, and underlying fascia to move upward as a unit.

2 The concept of high-sutured orbicularis oculi support to deep temporal fascia and/or periosteum alone, i.e., to hold up the lid or prevent ectropion, may deny the fact that the lid margin itself offers very little support. Thus, e.g., for festoons or full-cheek elevation, separate points of attachment along the lower rim and malar bone may also be crucial, not just at the new lid level or higher.

3 Motor innervation to the lower lid enters obliquely from the lateral off the temporal branch of VII, but primarily from below off the zygomatic branches of cranial nerve VII. Thus, the concept of a skin/muscle flap to leave innervated muscle is true, but it alone cannot support the entire lid and cheek.

4 The skin of the lid is very thin and the muscle of the lid is very vascular, with tremendous numbers of anastomoses. Thus, not only will full-thickness grafts of lid skin survive, but grafts of lid and muscle will also. This vascularity will also allow long, thin myocutaneous flaps to be transposed with success.

5 Surgeons have little problem approaching the orbital bones by many routes or the lateral wall, e.g., by orbitotomy or from above. Even the roof can be exposed, when required, by craniotomy or via a trans-lid approach. The medial orbital has not received enough "exposure," so the canalicular/fornix approach is presented. Note that the medial orbit can also be approached via a vertically oriented W in the medial upper lid, and otolaryngologists often utilize endoscopy for trans-sinus placement of support for the lamina papyracea.

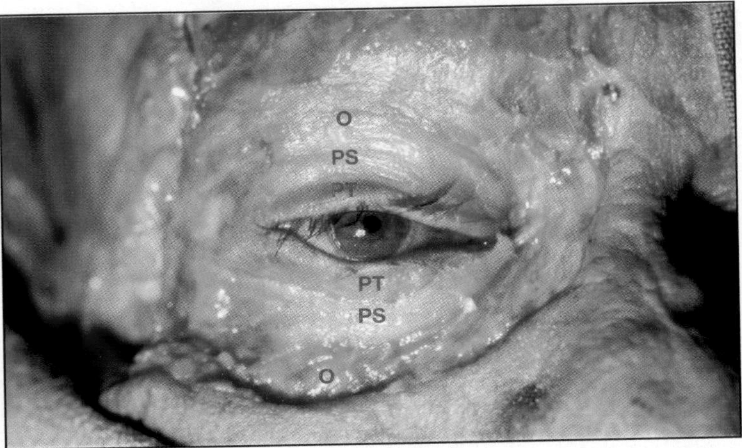

Figure 7D.1

The periorbital skin has been removed, exposing the orbicularis oculi muscle. This muscle acts as an antagonist to the levator palpebrae superioris muscle innervated by the third cranial nerve.

The orbicularis oculi muscle is divided into palpebral and orbital portions. The palpebral portion is further subdivided into pretarsal (PT) and preseptal (PS) portions.

The orbital portion (O) of the orbicularis oculi arises medially from the superomedial orbital margin, the maxillary process of the frontal bone, the medial canthal tendon, the frontal process of the maxilla, and the inferomedial orbital margin. The peripheral fibers sweep across the eyelid over the orbital margin in a series of concentric loops, the more central ones forming almost complete rings. In the upper lid, the orbital portion spreads upward onto the forehead, covers the corrugator supercilii muscle, and continues laterally over the anterior temporalis fascia. In the lower lid, the orbital portion covers the origins of the elevator muscles of the upper lip and nasal ala and continues temporally to cover part of the origin of the masseter muscle. Occasionally, the lower orbital portion interspersed with fat may actually continue downward into the cheek. The preseptal portion diverges from its origin on the medial canthal tendon and lacrimal diaphragm and passes across the lid as a series of half ellipses to meet at the later canthal raphe. The muscle bundles are not interrupted and do not interdigitate at the raphe. Medially, the orbicularis oculi unites to join the medial canthal tendon, which inserts on the medial orbital margin and nasal bones.

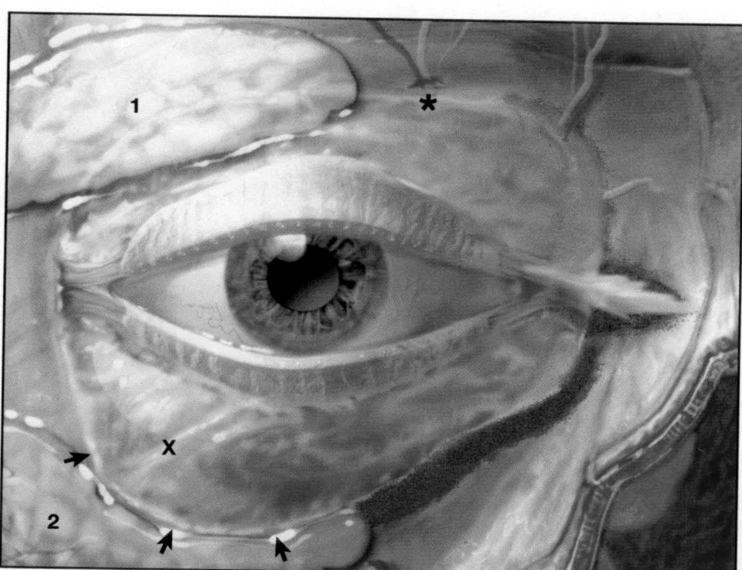

Figure 7D.2

The green outline denotes the medial origins of the orbicularis oculi muscle. The orbital septum is a fascial membrane that separates the eyelid structures from the deeper orbital structures.

The orbital septum attaches to the orbital margin at a thickening called the arcus marginalis (*arrows*). The arcus marginalis is also the point of confluence for the facial bone periosteum and the periorbita. The orbital septum is usually thicker *laterally* in both lids and thicker in the younger patient. Although the attachment follows the orbital margin for the most part, some key anatomic points must be made. First, laterally, the orbital septum lies in front of the lateral canthal tendon (although this is disputed). Second, superomedially, the arcus marginalis often forms the inferior part of the supraorbital groove (*). Therefore, the supraorbital neurovascular structures frequently exit from a groove or notch closed by the arcus marginalis. Third, medially, the orbital septum passes in front of the superior oblique trochlear pulley and then runs backward behind the deep heads of the orbicularis oculi onto the posterior lacrimal crest. Fourth, the orbital septum follows the rim along the inferior portion of the anterior lacrimal crest and inferior orbital rim. Finally, in the lateral half of the inferior orbital rim, the orbital septum actually originates a few millimeters inferior to the temporal orbital margin, forming a potential space on the facial aspect of the zygoma (the recess of Eisler).

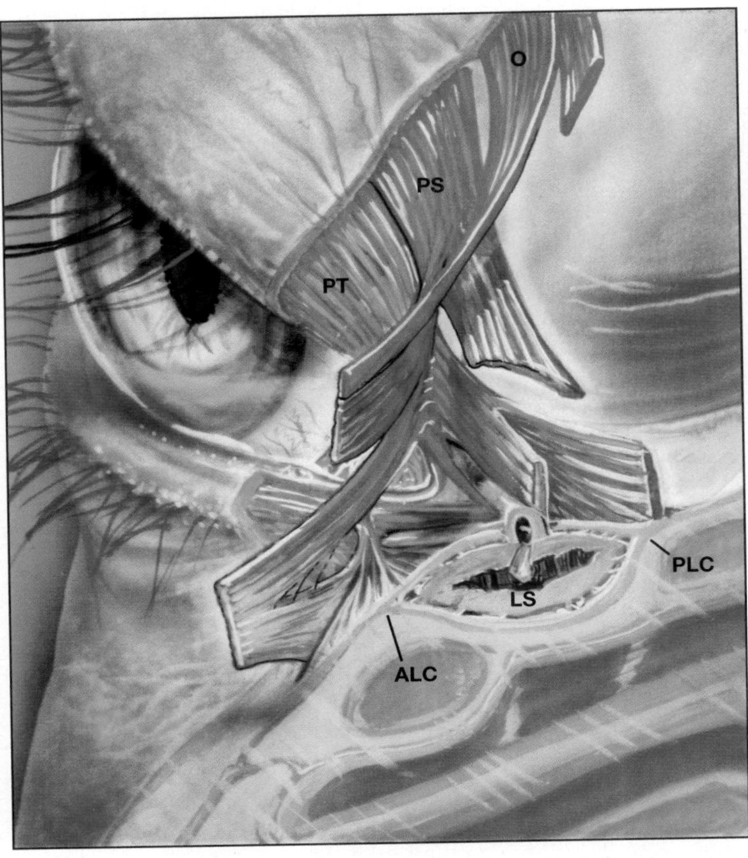

Figure 7D.3

The nose has been cut away to show the origins of the orbicularis oculi fibers and their relation to the lacrimal sac (LS). The anterior component of the medial canthal tendon extends forward anterior to the sac. The palpebral portion of the orbicularis oculi muscle can be separated into pretarsal (PT) and preseptal (PS) components. Furthermore, these components possess deep and superficial heads as they pass medially. The deeper fibers pass posteriorly to the lacrimal sac and its fascia and to the posterior lacrimal crest, and they are vital to proper lacrimal pump function. The deeper pretarsal fibers have been termed *Horner's muscle*, the *pars lacrimalis*, or *tensor tarsi*. Note that the medial canthal tendon extends beyond the anterior lacrimal crest (ALC) to the frontal process of the maxilla. The orbital portion of the orbicularis oculi fibers (O) arises from the medial orbital margin, as noted previously.

The orbital septum passes in front of the superior oblique pulley, then runs back behind the deep heads of the orbicularis oculi onto the posterior lacrimal crest. The transcaruncular (with or without the fornix) approach to the medial requires understanding this anatomy.

The medial wall may be approached via a transcaruncular method, which can be extended into the lower fornix if necessary. The caruncle, that soft tissue fold just inside the canthus, is retracted while 5 mL of local anesthetic is injected there and into the medial orbital region along the wall. A lateral, slightly curved (12-mm vertical) caruncular splitting incision is made, which can be enlarged by Stevens scissors toward the posterior lacrimal crest. The orbital septum is kept laterally. The retractors can be placed and the incision lengthened if necessary. A needle cautery is used to cut through periorbita to expose bone (see 7D.4).

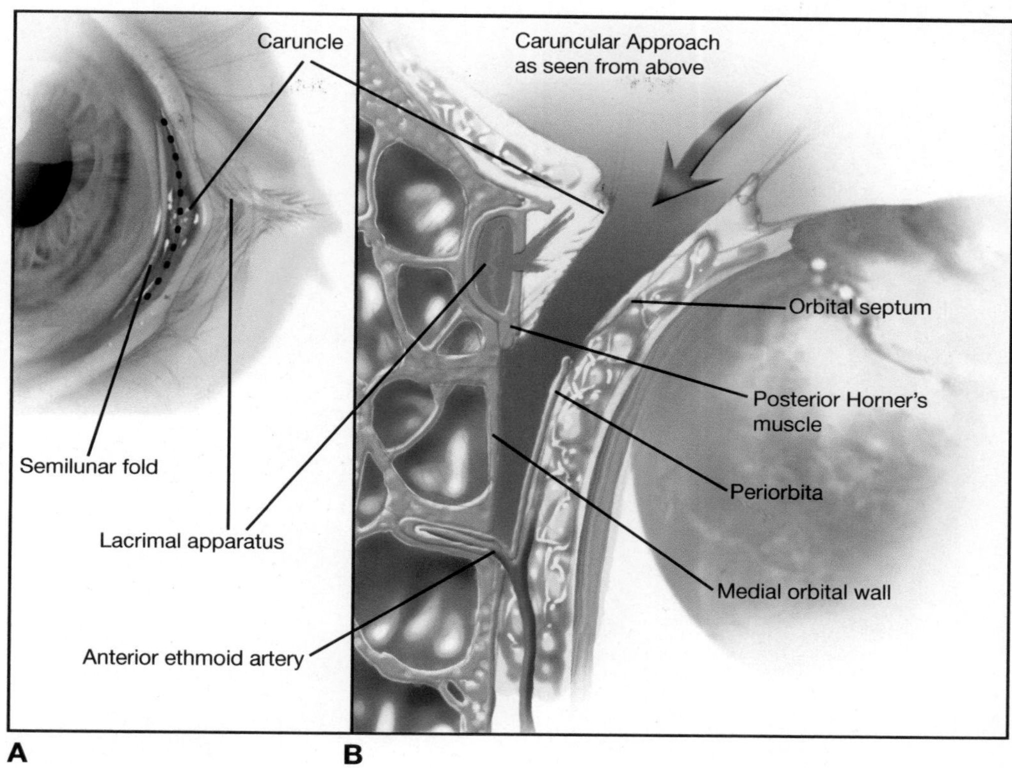

Figure 7D.4A–B

The fascia deep to the caruncle is continuous with the medial canthal tendon. The medial fascia is the anterior insertion of Horner's muscle, the anterior part of Tenon's capsule, and the medial orbital septum. The medial orbital septum inserts into the periorbita behind the posterior lacrimal crest along with Horner's muscle. The scissors are opened tangentially passing through the avascular plane between Horner's muscle and the medial orbital septum posterior to the lacrimal crest. This is a natural plane to the medial orbit, and if the fornix is also opened, great exposure can be obtained. Closure is simple with a 6-0 plain suture.

Note: When the fornix approach is combined with the caruncular approach, the inferior oblique muscle may require disinsertion from the floor, and this can be replaced later. Diplopia does not occur postoperatively with proper repositioning of the muscle.

Data column—Key facts.

1. The anterior ethmoidal canal (with nerve and artery) is 20 mm behind the anterior orbital margin, and the posterior canal is 12 mm behind that. The anterior ethmoidal artery and nerve enter the anterior cranial fossa and then, via the cribriform plate, reach the nose.
2. The anterior ethmoidal nerve (off the nasociliary) supplies mucosa of the anterior ethmoidal air cells and mucosa of the upper anterior nose, then proceeds to the nasal tip. Herpes zoster that affects this nerve may present at the nasal tip (Hutchinson's sign).
3. The medial wall is the thinnest, and the lateral wall the thickest.

CHAPTER 7e

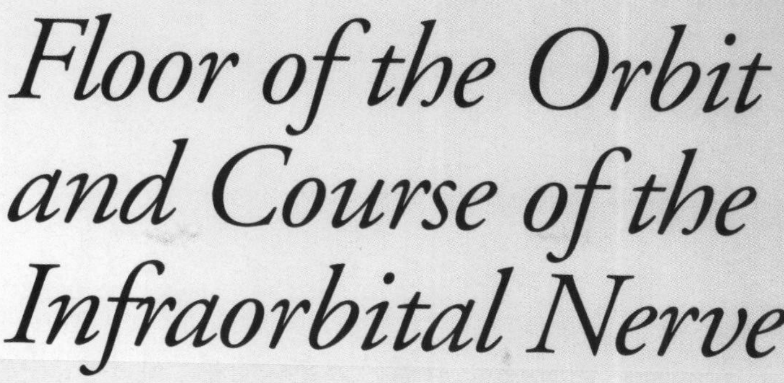

Floor of the Orbit and Course of the Infraorbital Nerve

1 The zygomatic branch of the maxillary nerve leaves the infraorbital branch soon after the entrance to the inferior orbital fissure.

2 The zygomatic branch separates into zygomaticofacial and zygomaticotemporal branches, as seen previously.

3 The infraorbital nerve passes below a thin central orbital floor, passing more medially to come out at the infraorbital foramen.

4 Prior to the exit, the infraorbital nerve has two or three branches to the ipsilateral teeth and gingiva; these are the posterior and middle superior alveolar nerves and the anterior superior alveolar nerve, which comes off 5 to 20 mm prior to the foramen. The posterior branch is back much further and requires injection behind the maxillary tuberosity where it enters the bone.

An injection directly into the foramen may also affect the anterior superior alveolar nerve (see Chapter 8).

5 Direct injection of the infraorbital nerve does not lead to neuritis, but the patient may get a quick electric shock sensation there, if the needle hits the nerve directly.

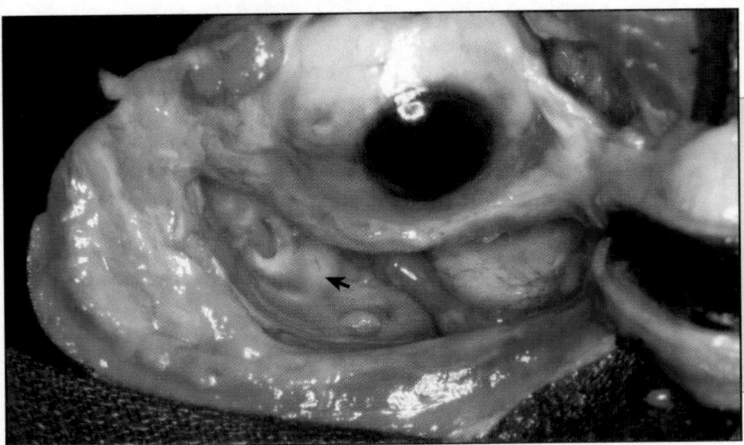

Figure 7E.1A

The upper and lower eyelids have been detached from the lateral orbital tubercle and reflected medially. The orbital fat has been removed, exposing the inferior orbit.

The inferior oblique muscle has been said to separate the medial lower lid compartment from the lateral region. The infraorbital nerve is visible below the thin orbital floor (*arrow*).

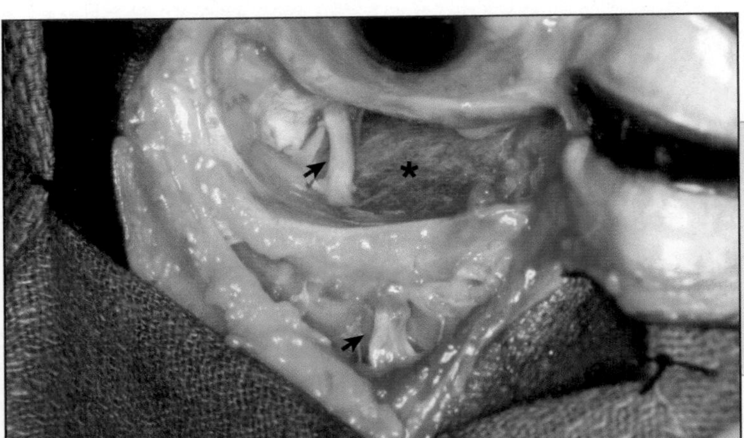

B

Figure 7E.1B

Part of the bony floor of the orbit has been removed, exposing the maxillary sinus mucosa (*) and infraorbital nerve (*arrow*). Note that the nerve courses from a lateral position to its more medially located infraorbital foramen in line with the medial limbus on the anterior face of the maxilla.

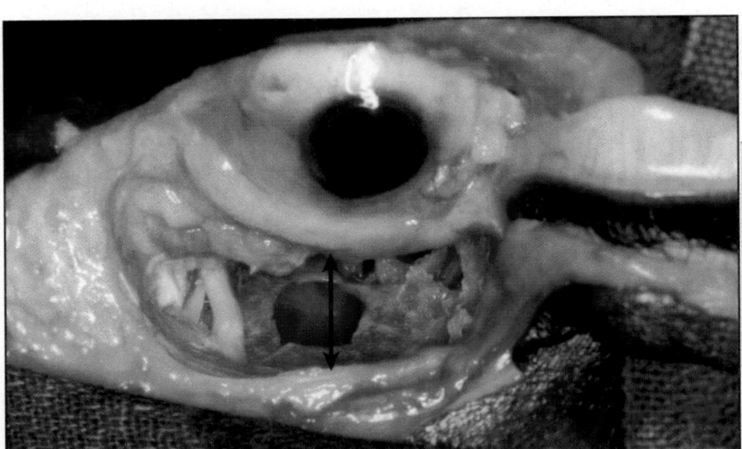

C

Figure 7E.1C

A hole has been made in the mucosa to expose the sinus. Note that this dissection is at least 35 mm back and still quite safe. The posterior safe distance along the floor is about 40 mm back, as the optic foramen is about 50 mm in men and slightly less in women (see Chapter 1).

Figure 7E.2

The infraorbital nerve is seen exiting the infraorbital foramen. The foramen, approximately 4 mm in diameter, opens in an *inferior or inferior and medial orientation*. The foramen is approximately 5 to 8 mm below the infraorbital margin. A needle directed to enter the foramen for a nerve block should be placed through the skin medial to the upper aspect of the nasolabial fold to be in the correct direction.

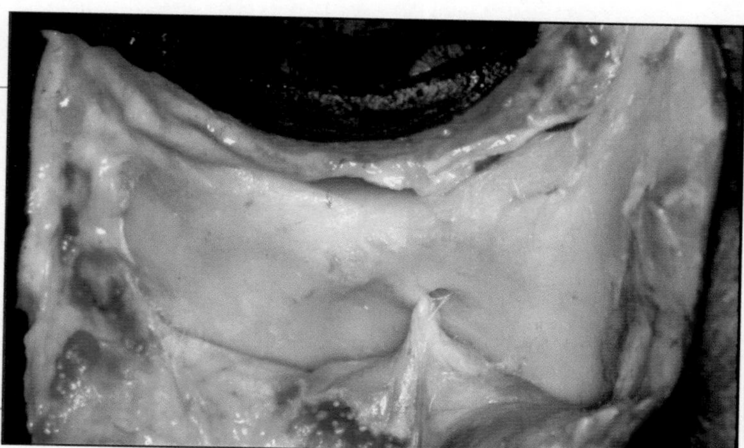

Figure 7E.3

A piece of bone has been removed below the medial orbital rim. The very red maxillary sinus mucosa can be seen. Medial to this the nasolacrimal duct traverses downward to exit below the inferior turbinate. The exit point in the nose has a valve (the valve of Hasner) that prevents mucosa from entering the eyelid fornix during nose blowing.

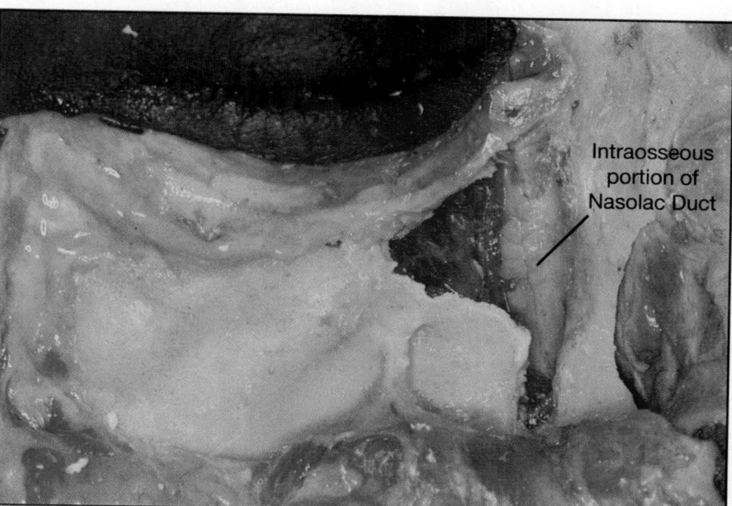

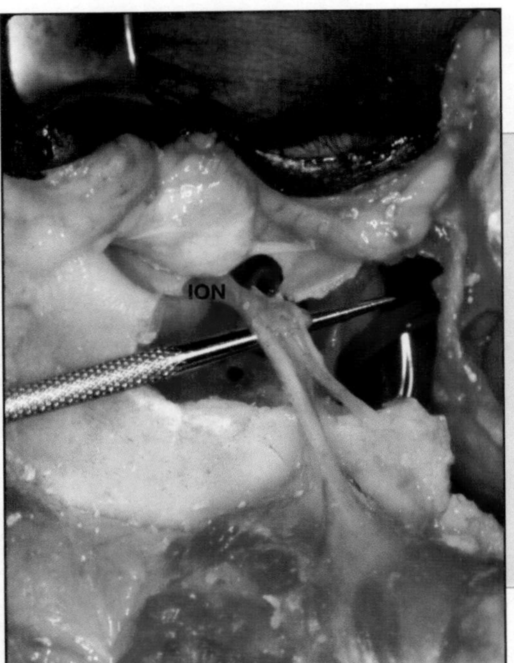

Figure 7E.4

The anterior maxilla has been cleared of muscle to expose the infraorbital nerve (ION). Maxillary bone removal medial and superior to the nerve exposes the underlying maxillary sinus. Note the anterior superior alveolar nerve, which comes off between 5 and 20 mm prior to the exit of the ION. This nerve passes through the *canalis spinosus* in the maxillary face to supply sensation to the anterior gingiva and front four teeth on that side. Thus, a fracture of the medial maxillary face or a medially placed Caldwell-Luc approach may desensitize the front four teeth and gingiva.

CHAPTER 7f

Intranasal

The purpose of these dissections relates to two subjects:

1 The relation and course of the nasolacrimal apparatus into the nose.

2 How to perform a sphenopalatine (pterygopalatine) ganglion block, which accomplish the following:
—Reduces tear production.
—Blocks mucosa of the posterior superior and middle conchae, the nasal septum, the roof of the nasal cavity, and much of the nasal floor forward to the incisor foramen.
—Numbs the palate (hard and soft).

2a The opening for the nerve behind the middle turbinate can also be approached by a "cocainized" pledget placed 7 to 8 cm inside the nose. The exact placement of this anesthetic pledget is usually difficult because of the turbinate size and anatomic variations.

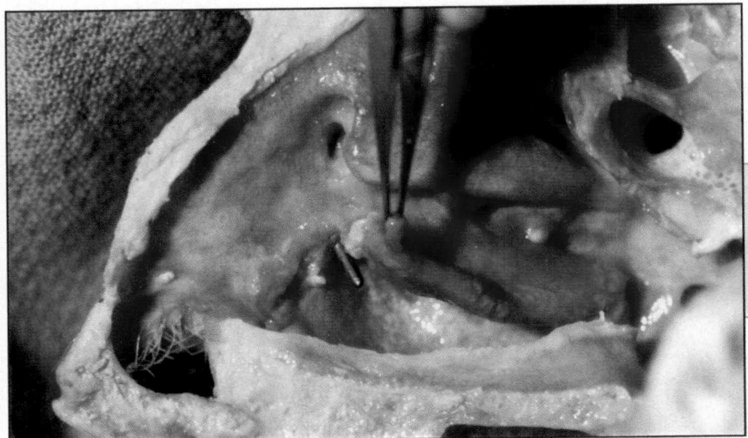

Figure 7F.1

A probe is passed from the lacrimal sac region into the nose to exit under the front of the inferior turbinate. The turbinate has been released anteriorly to show this.

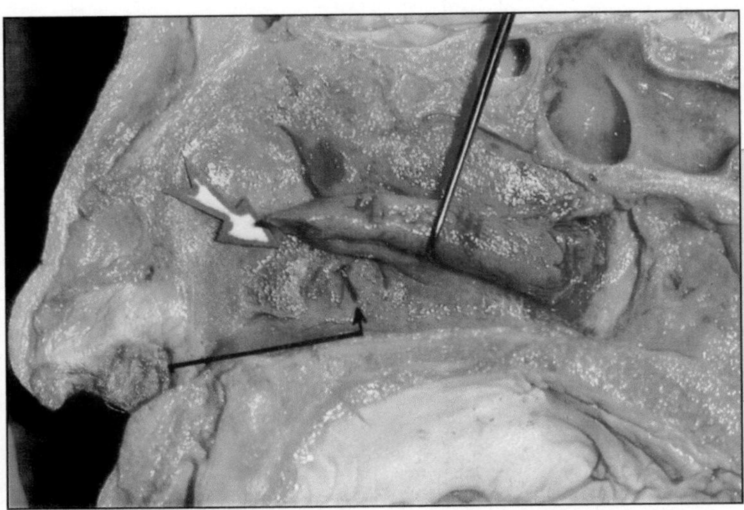

Figure 7F.2

The inferior turbinate is incised anteriorly (*blue arrow*) and reflected upward. The probe exits the slit valve (of Hasner) as noted, approximately 40 mm from the opening of the nose. This valve prevents mucus from going into the eye during nose blowing. An incompetent valve will allow mucus to exit the puncta in some patients.

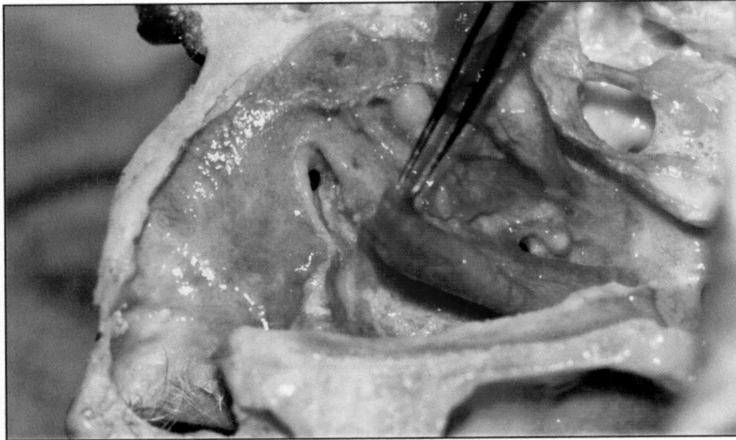

Figure 7F.3

The length of this canal is usually about 1.8 cm and is directed back about 15 degrees in this specimen where the bone has been removed. Thus, tubes or catheters threaded through the puncta would exit here at the inferior meatus for later removal.

Figure 7F.4

Surgeons who perform cleft palate work know where the greater palatine foramen is in the child. In the adult (*lower arrow*), it is usually found a centimeter or so medial and posterior to the junction of the first and second molars or posterior to that, between the second and third. The surgeon should use a 25-gauge bent needle on a small syringe with a little local anesthetic to find it exactly. The needle is usually bent at a 60-degree angle or greater, and the foramen can be found easily. The upper arrow points to the posterior middle turbinate

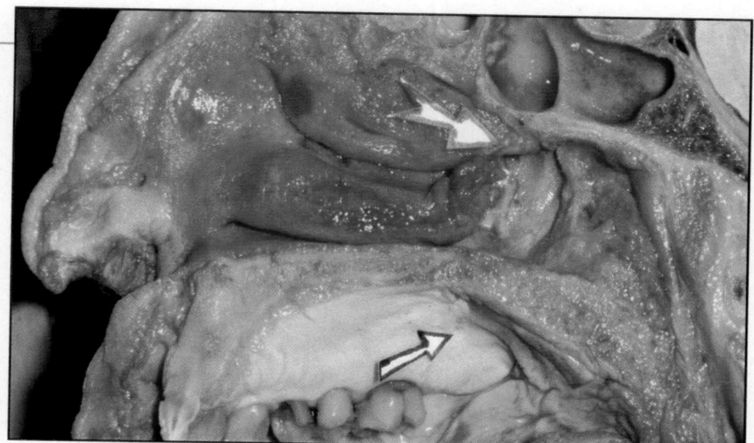

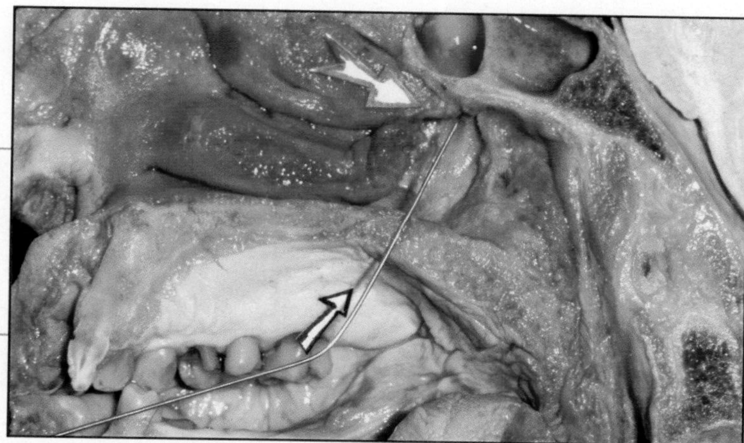

Figure 7F.5

A 22-gauge spinal needle is then bent so that no greater than 4 to 4.5 cm can be put into the greater palatine foramen. The canal does angle back a little, but the surgeon's finger on the needle bend will advance it.

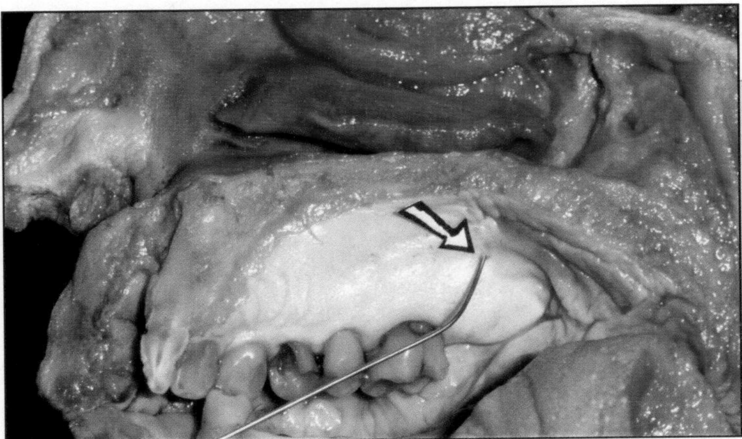

Figure 7F.6

In this case, the needle was advanced just over 4 cm to hit the area of nerve exiting the lateral nasal wall. Because the ganglion is above this nerve exit, it is usually safe to inject higher (~0.5 cm), but not necessary. The author has found that a 1½-in. needle will not work, but going about a centimeter farther works well as you have to accommodate for oral mucosal thickness and the needle's bend.

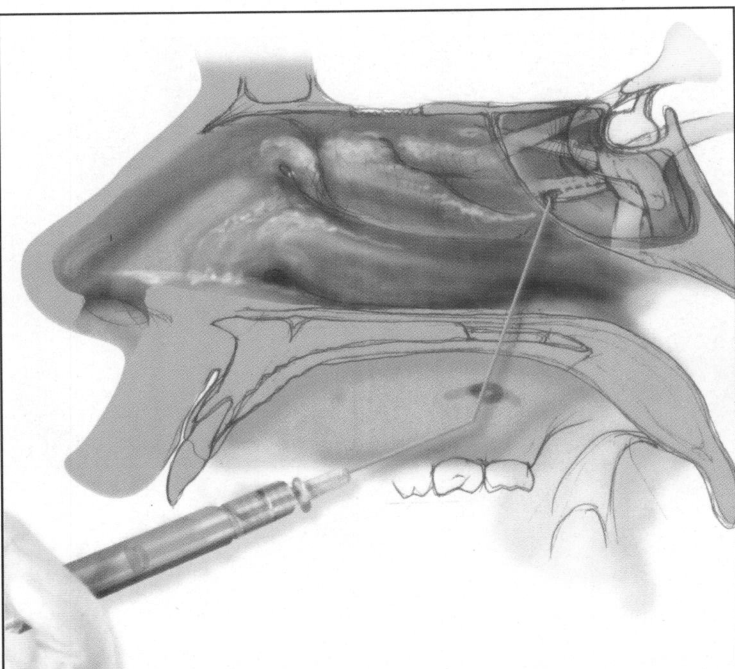

Figure 7F.7

Schematic of the block.

CHAPTER 8

Nerve Blocks 101

In a 1998 article titled "How to Block and Tackle the Face"[1], I presented a system for facile nerve blocks that would allow the surgeon to be more effective and efficient with local anesthesia once the block methods were adopted. I did not show the intraoral injections (e.g., inferior alveolar nerve or the long buccal nerve course) that I use, since most nondental surgeons shy away from them. In a like manner, I avoided intraorbital blocks used by ophthalmologists. In this chapter, I have made some additions, namely, for the lacrimal nerve (which I originally omitted) and for the cervical plexus, which will extend the surgeon's range to the neck. Furthermore, as I am not constrained by journal limitations, the exposition is much grander in photographs and schematics and, thus, easier to understand.

My fervent hope for all who read this chapter is that you immediately start to practice these blocks. Once you become proficient, you will never again directly inject the nasal tip or lip without blocking first because you will know how much it will hurt. You will block the lips in preparation for marking the white roll with needles dipped in ink. You will start performing cases with blocks and simple oral premedications and marvel at your own skills.

[1]Zide BM, Swift R. How to block and tackle the face. *Plast. Reconstr. Surg.* 1998;101(3):840–851.

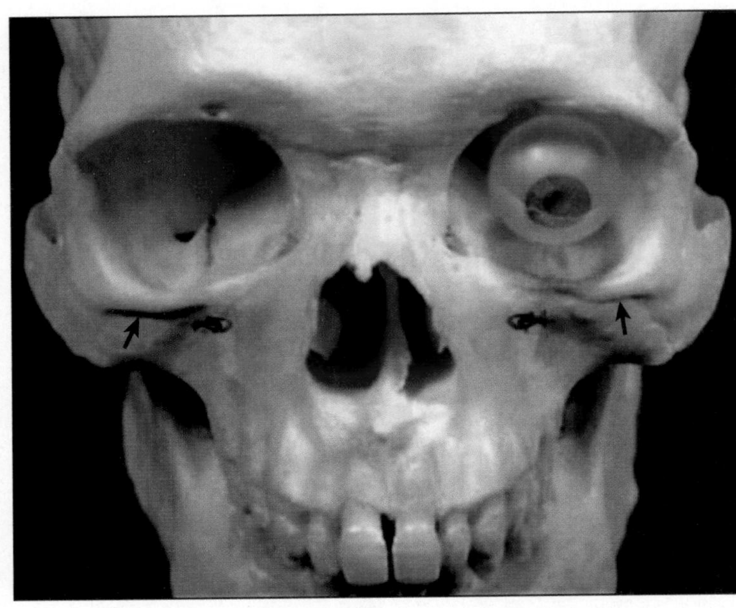

Figure 8.1

The infraorbital nerve opens downward and medially above 5–8 mm below the rim. In some cases the lower rim may have a ridge (*arrows*) which may be mistaken for fracture.

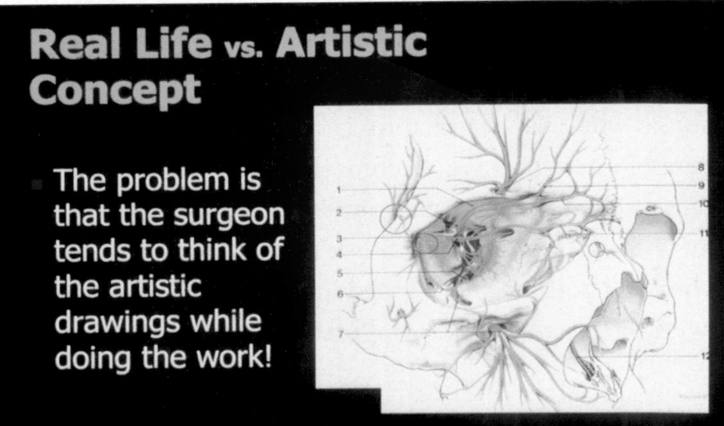

Figure 8.2

My original article[1] explained block techniques to anesthetize the entire face. Some things were left out, but the overall explanation found there makes solid reading.

As anatomy is taught less and less, we have learned to rely on illustrators' drawings. If they are wrong, how can we think correctly in the operating room? The red circled areas in this drawing by a first class artist shows nerves going in incorrect directions and in incorrect positions.

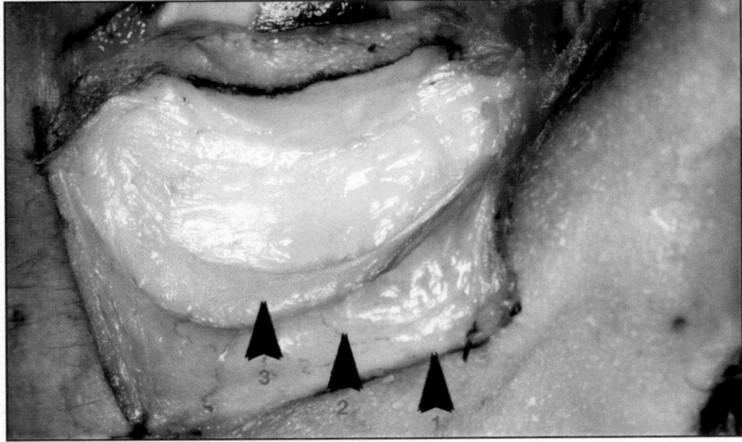

Figure 8.3

Where is the infraorbital nerve on straight gaze? Under 1, 2, or 3? Most people choose no. 2, but the answer is no. 1, on a line dropped from the medial limbus.

The distance from the rim to the foramen is slightly greater for men, but 5.5 to 7.5 ± ½ mm is the range.

[1] Reprinted with permission from Eriksson, E. Illustrated Handbook in Local Anesthesia. Philadelphia: W.B. Saunders, 1980;59.

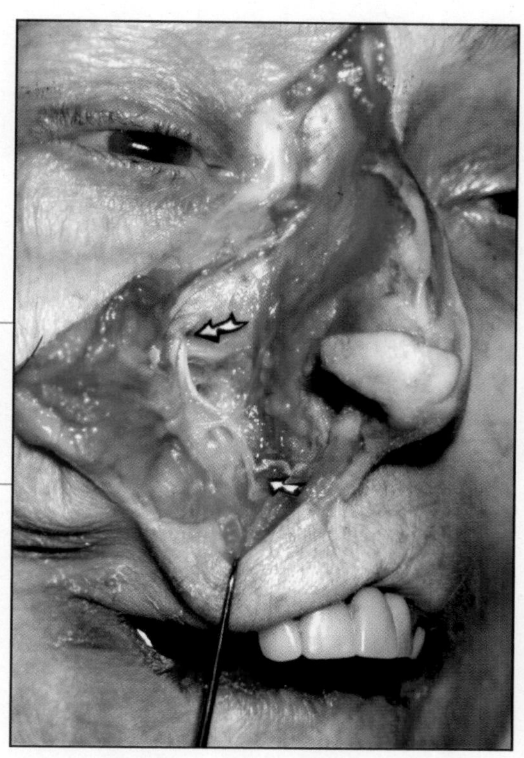

Figure 8.4

- The upper arrow shows the infraorbital exit.
- The lower arrow shows a distal branch that rides over the levator to the upper lip to supply the *base of the columella.*

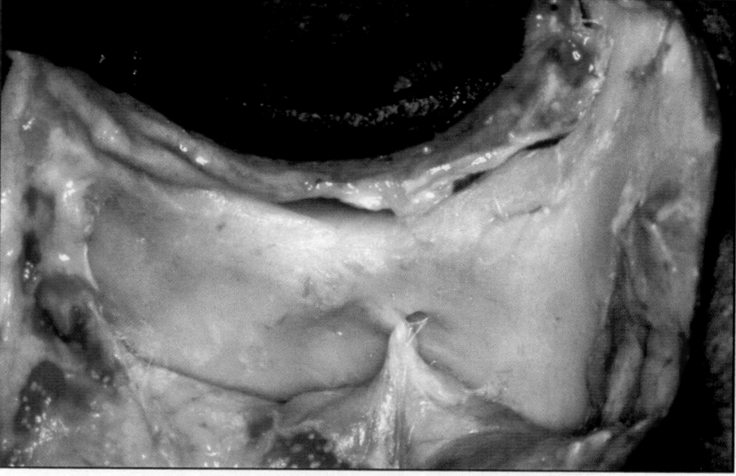

Figure 8.5

The foramen opens downward and medially, so injections to it should come from below and medial.

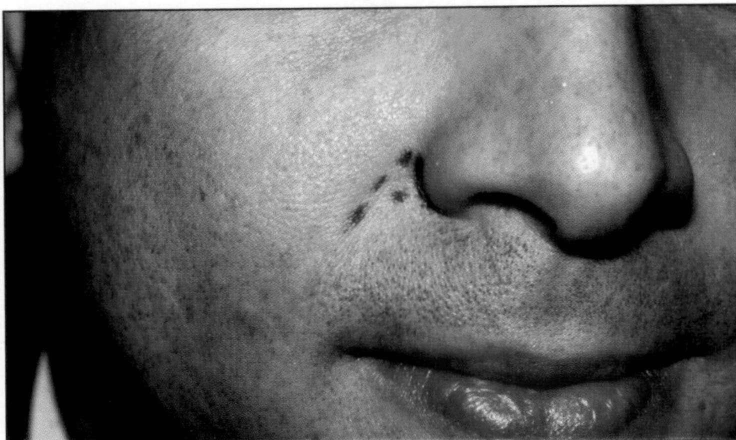

Figure 8.6

The dot between the nasolabial fold and alar base is the best entrance point.

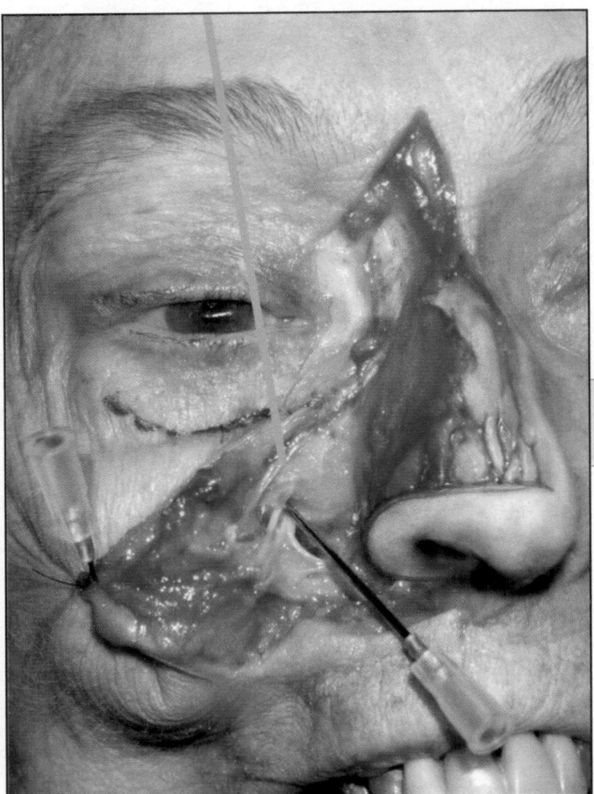

Figure 8.7

The rim is marked in green. The foramen is 5 to 8 mm down on a line from the medial limbus.

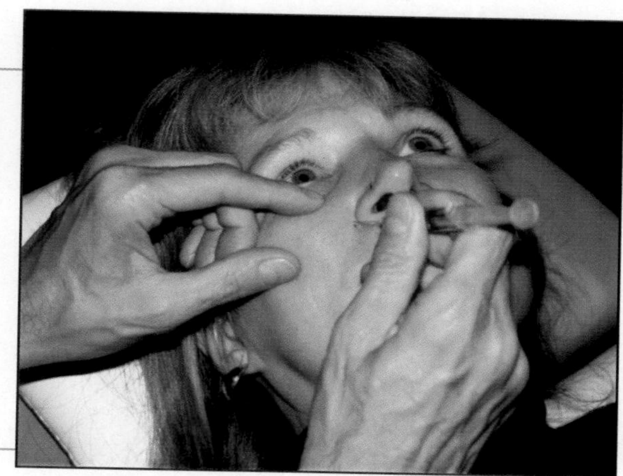

Figure 8.8

With a finger on the rim, the patient looks forward. The needle is held with a *pen grip*, and the surgeon inserts the needle to the foramen. With little practice, the surgeon can get into the foramen 90% of the time, and that number increases.

Tell the patient he or she may feel an electric shock; that's good a sign. At that point, you should inject because your position is correct. You will never get a neuritis.

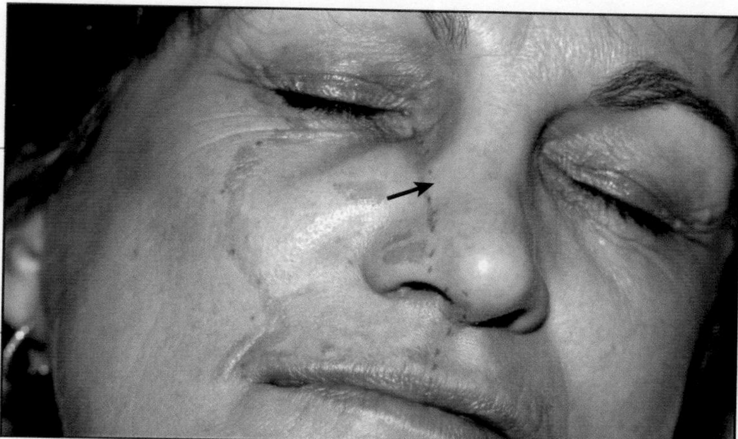

Figure 8.9

This zone is the usual area of numbness for this block. Often, though, the numbness encroaches more on the lip or sidewall of the nose. In addition the lateral red border may often cover a larger area.

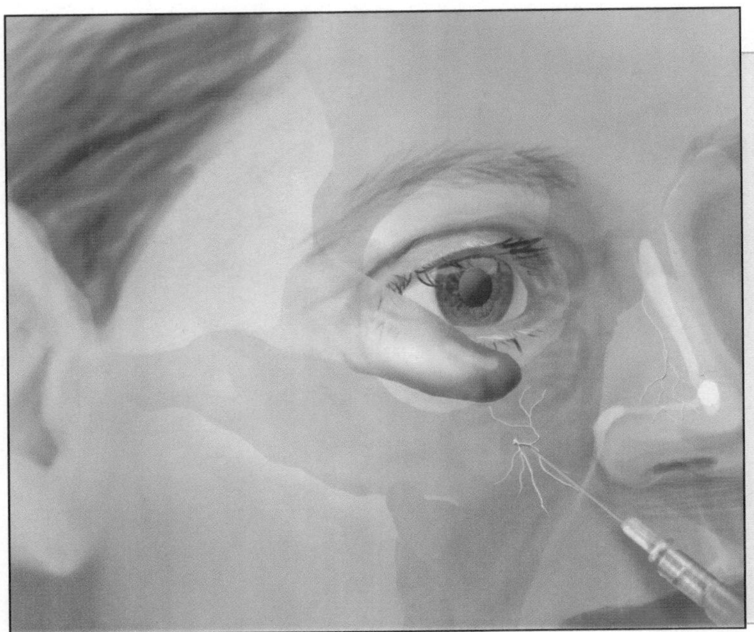

Figure 8.10

If the needle enters the foramen, the anterior superior alveolar nerve—which comes off between 5 and 20 mm prior to the foramen—may be blocked. In that case, the gingiva and front four teeth on that side will be affected.

The anterior superior alveolar nerve travels through a small canal in the anterior maxilla (canalis spinosus) before supplying the teeth. Therefore, if the maxillary face is fractured, yet the lip has normal sensation and the gingiva is numb, the anterior face of the maxilla may be cracked.

At times, a Caldwell-Luc opening to the maxillary sinus will desensitize the teeth and gingiva ipsilaterally due to disruption of the intrabony course of the anterior superior alveolar nerve.

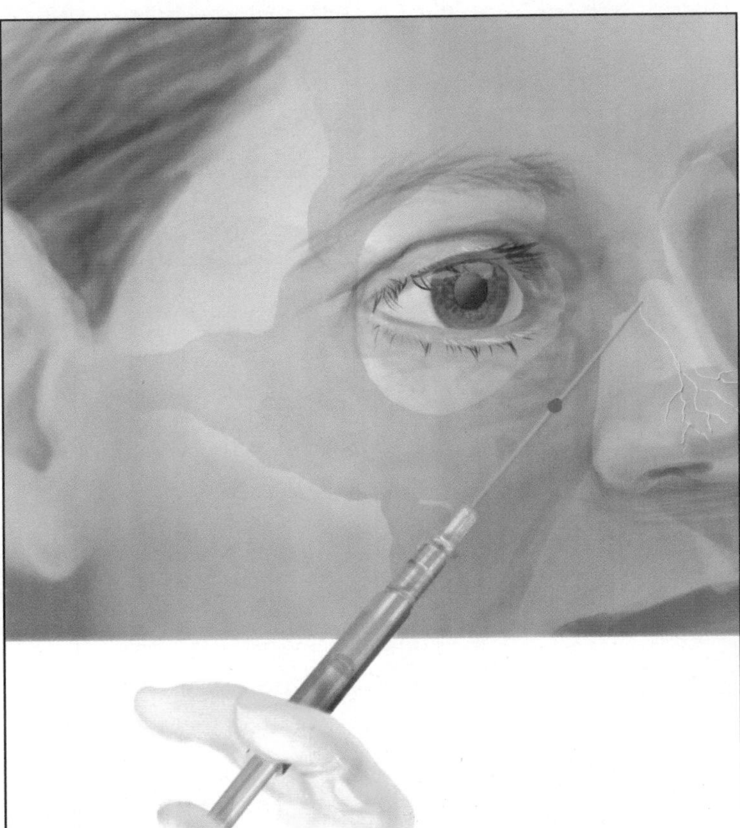

Figure 8.11

The dorsal nasal nerve, the dorsal branch(es) of the ethmoidal nerve, exits from under the nasal bone edge about 6 to 9 mm from the midline. There may be 1–3 branches although only one is shown. It passes under the nasalis muscle and provides sensation to the nasal tip. Once the infraorbital nerve is blocked, the dorsal nasal nerve can be blocked with a painless stick. The dorsal nasal nerve may have one to three branches to the tip region.

Clinically, for a nasal tip lesion, the skin's adherence to underlying cartilage makes direct injection painful. Blocking prior to tip injection is always a better option.

Figure 8.12

Transection of the nerve(s) is common via an intercartilaginous nasal incision, which explains tip numbness after some rhinoplasties.

This block can be done from above or from the side, gliding along the deep distal bony edge toward or from the cheek after your infraorbital injection has been done. Where it comes out depends on nasal bone length to some degree. As it passes through a small groove at the edge of the nasal bones, it may remain single or split.

The dorsal nasal nerve exits between 6.5 and 8.5 cm from the midline under the nasalis muscles (i.e., under the nasal SMAS layer). Anywhere from one to three branches may be found coursing almost straight along the midline toward the nasal tip.

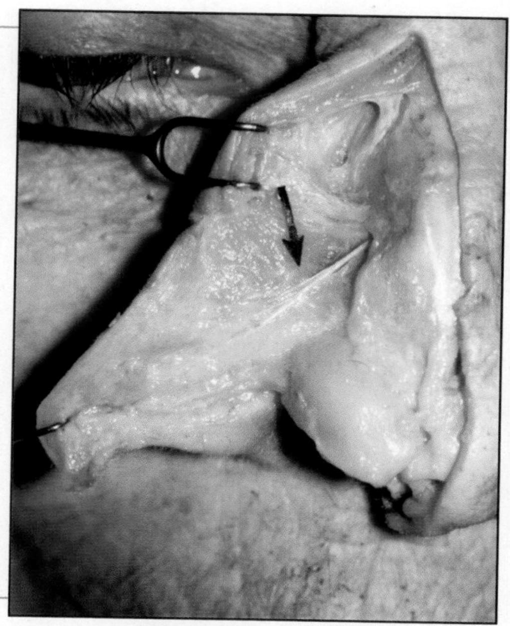

Figure 8.13

Top: Dental professionals are taught early on the method of blocking the inferior alveolar nerve as it enters the lingula on the medial surface of the ramus. In addition, the long buccal nerve may be injected behind the third molar along the lower ramus, which will affect the cheek. Some physicians—e.g., some surgical dermatologists, plastic surgeons, and otolaryngologists—may feel better operating more toward the surface.

The sensation of the entire lower lip from commissure to commissure depends on blocking the mental nerves. Usually three or four branches exit the mental foramen about the apex of the first or second bicuspids, but this varies. The 2–3 lip branches that block from the labiomental fold to vermilion can be effaced with the thumb for easy visualization. A third branch, and sometimes others through bone, supplies sensation to the chin pad; however, in many cases, a sensory branch off the mylohyoid nerve supplies a quarter-sized area of the chin pad on each side. Therefore, the pad will need additional supraperiosteal injection, as will be shown.

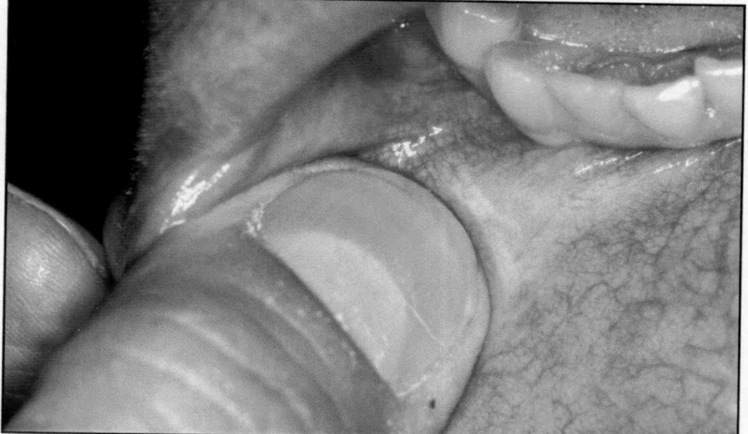

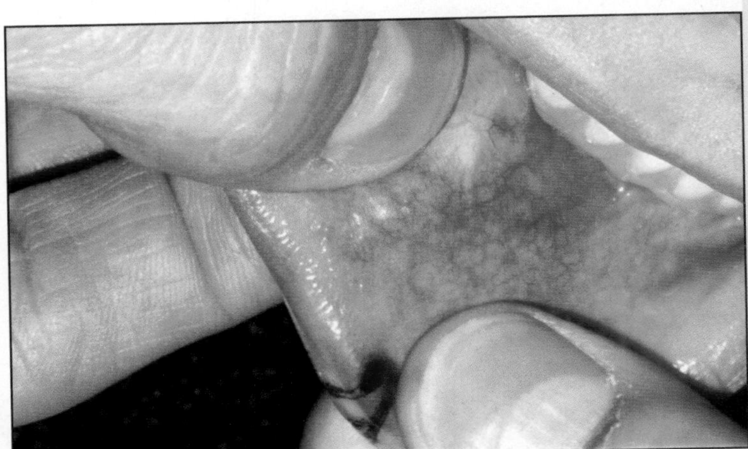

Figures 8.14

With thumb pressure down and lateral, the mental nerves' superior branches can be found from 5 to 10 mm away from the canine. A few drops of local anesthetic under the mucosa here will often, but not always, block the lower lip. Occasionally, because of early branching, you may need to add a little under the mucosa a bit more distally. Among people with darker skin, the darker mucosa may make visualization harder, yet after a while the position just lateral to the canine becomes fixed in your mind. For consistent, more extensive coverage of the chin pad, the surgeon must do the mental plus (M+) injections.

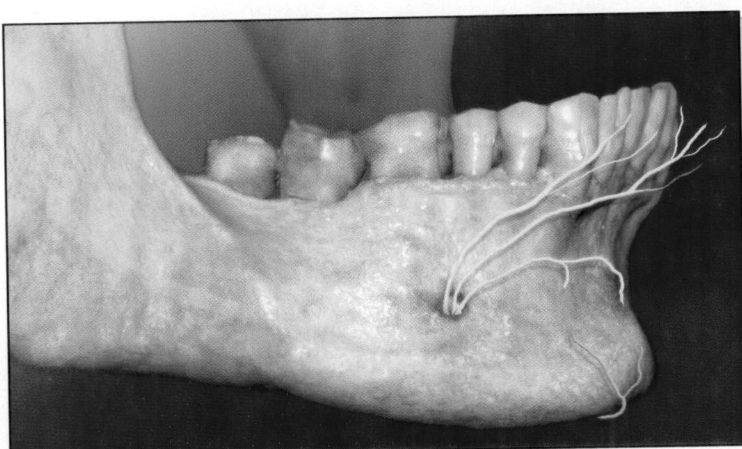

Figure 8.15

The mental nerve exits the foramen usually as several fascicles. The top 2–3 may split early, or stay together and split while visible under the mucosa, as shown. Another branch, and perhaps one from the bone, supplies sensation to the chin pad. In many cases, a sensory branch off the mylohyoid nerve (*orange*) supplies a quarter-sized area of the ipsilateral pad. Therefore, after doing the submucosal block for the labiomental fold to and including vermilion, additional anesthesia will be required for the pad. The branch from the mylohyoid is noted in orange.

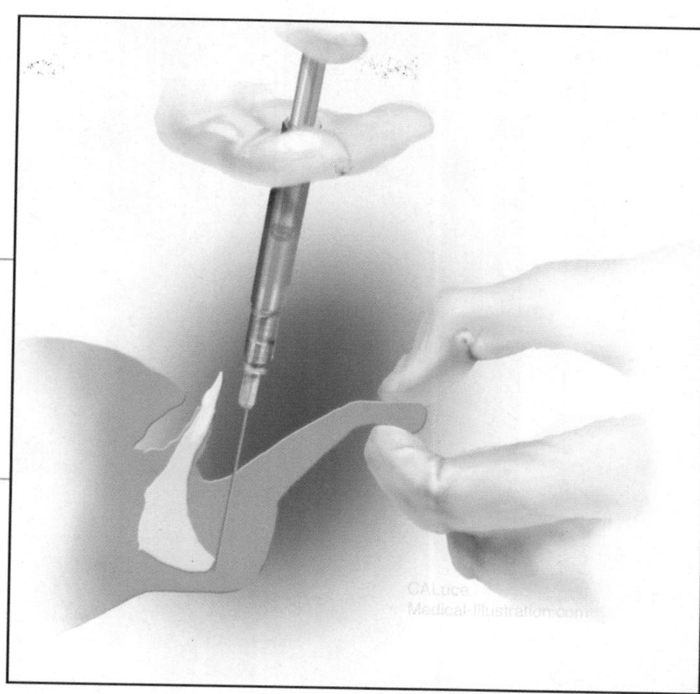

Figure 8.16

Standing above the patient, a 25- to 27-gauge, 1½-in. needle is passed through the lip (not the vestibule) to inject preperiosteally over a wide area, down almost to the submental dermis. With fanning injections from each side, surface or bony work can be performed.

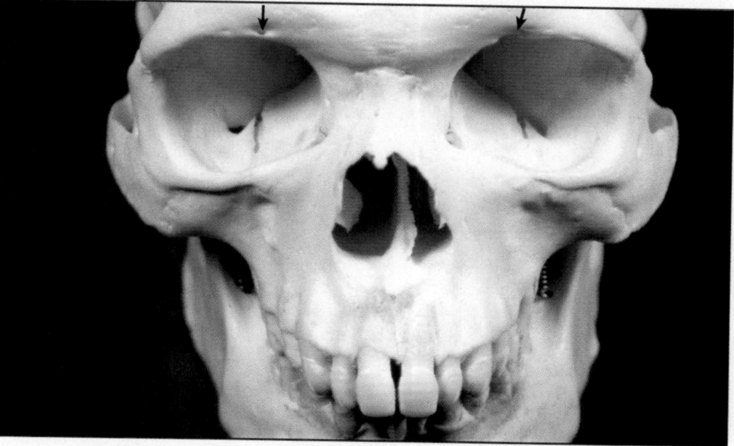

Figure 8.17

On the right side of the skull, the supraorbital nerve seems to exit a foramen, while on the left, a notch (*arrows*). The inferior part of the notch is the arcus marginalis, the periosteal confluence at the rim. Medial to the supraorbital nerves, which exit 2.2 to 2.9 cm from the midline, the supratrochlears come around the superomedial rim 1.5 to 2.2 cm from the midline. The infratrochlear nerves, which supply the upper nose and nasofrontal region, exit medially and inferiorly to that. Thus, to block these nerves, it would seem that the injection should come from lateral to medial along the rim toward the nasofrontal region.

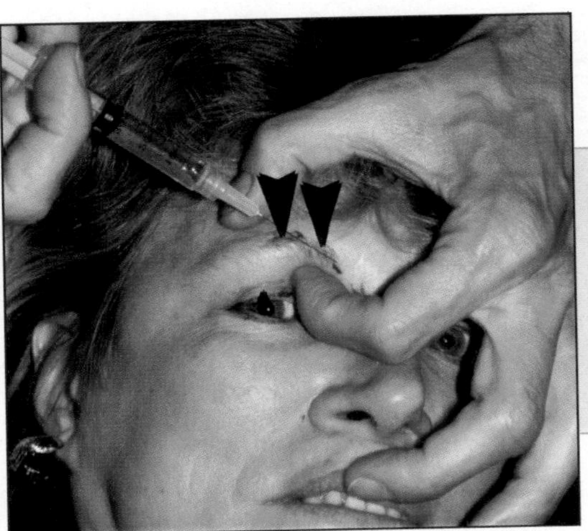

Figure 8.18

The needle direction is noted. The finger keeps feel of the needle as it passes along the rim to hit the nose. The needle (1½ in.) reaches the nasal bone. Remember to put pressure over the supraorbital region for a minute or two because of the veins there. A "black eye" is very common with this injection.

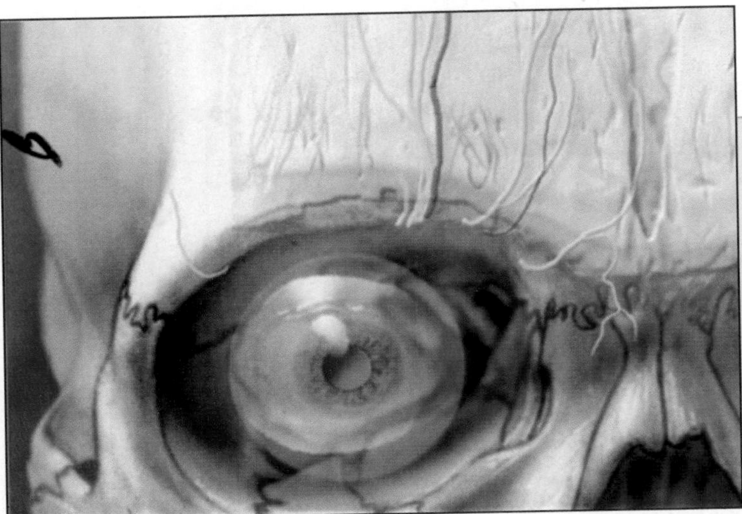

Figure 8.19

This block will affect three (and perhaps four if it gets the deep branch of the supraorbital) nerves: (1) supraorbital—medial branch, possibly the lateral or deep branch; (2) supratrochlear; and (3) infratrochlear—if the needle is passed all the way to the nasal bones. *Note:* The vein accompanying the supraorbital may result in ecchymosis if pressure is not applied postinjection.

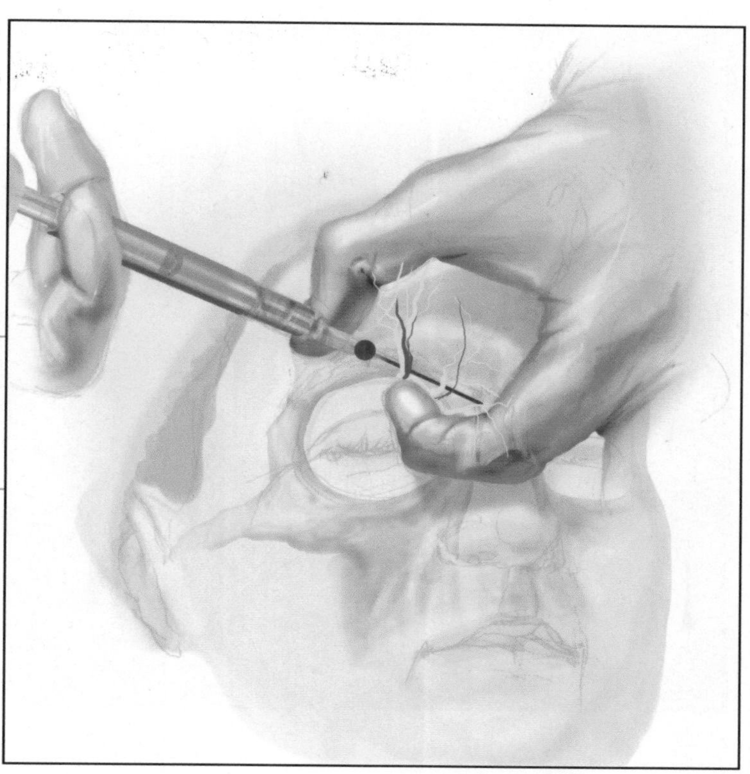

Figure 8.20

The needle is inserted about a cm or slightly more from the midline (over the lateral limbus) until it hits nasal bone. Inject 2 to 3 mL on the way out.

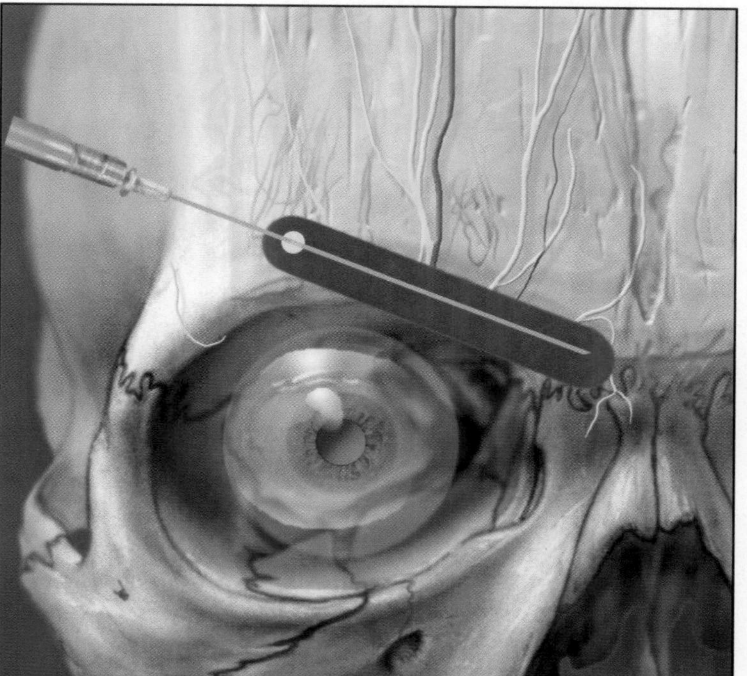

Figure 8.21

After 2 mL is deposited on exit, pressure is applied over the supraorbital notch/foramen area to decrease bruising. If the lateral branch comes from the same exit as the medial, the upper lateral forehead will be numb.

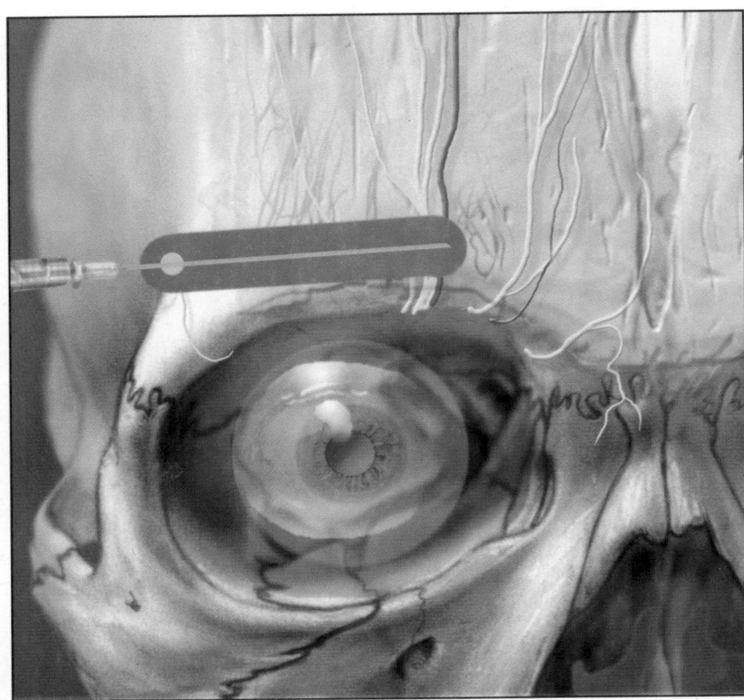

Figure 8.22

As the lateral (deep) branch may exit from 1 cm above the rim and up to 3 to 4 cm lateral to the medial branch, a submuscular deposit is made about 1 cm above the rim, as noted.

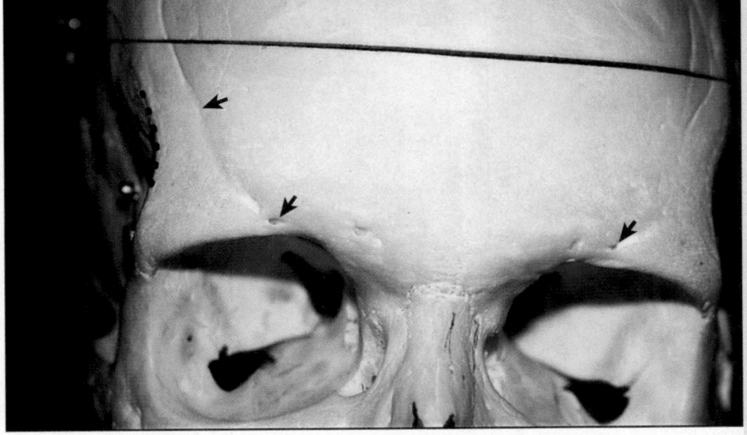

Figure 8.23

The supraorbital nerve has two key branches:

1. A medial or superficial branch, which goes through the frontalis muscle to be on top of the frontalis and to supply sensation to the bulk of the forehead and anterior scalp over the eyebrows.
2. A lateral or deep branch or branches (one to three), which travel supraperiosteally or, sometimes, under the periosteum. The lateral branch courses medial to the superior temporal line (*dotted*) and may exit in many ways: (a) with the medial branch; (b) through a close but separate foramen as seen here (*arrows*); (c) anywhere from above or to 3 to 4 cm later to the supraorbital notch/foramen.

These two skulls show the groove made by a subperiosteal branch along the correct course.

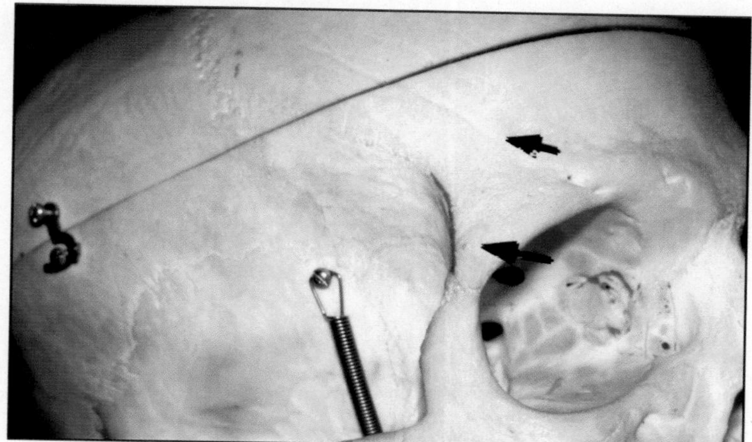

Figure 8.24

The supraorbital nerve from a different angle (repeated legend):

1. A medial or superficial branch, which goes through the frontalis muscle to be on top of the frontalis and to supply the bulk of the forehead and anterior scalp over the eyebrows.
2. A lateral or deep branch or branches (one to three), which travel supraperiosteally or, sometimes, under the periosteum. The lateral branch courses medial to the superior temporal line (*dotted*) and may exit in many ways: (a) with the medial branch; (b) through a close but separate foramen as seen here (*arrows*); (c) anywhere from above or to 3 to 4 cm later to the supraorbital notch/foramen.

This skull shows the groove made by a subperiosteal branch along the correct course. In this skull, a red line denotes the lower superior temporal line, and the arrow, as above, shows the course of travel.

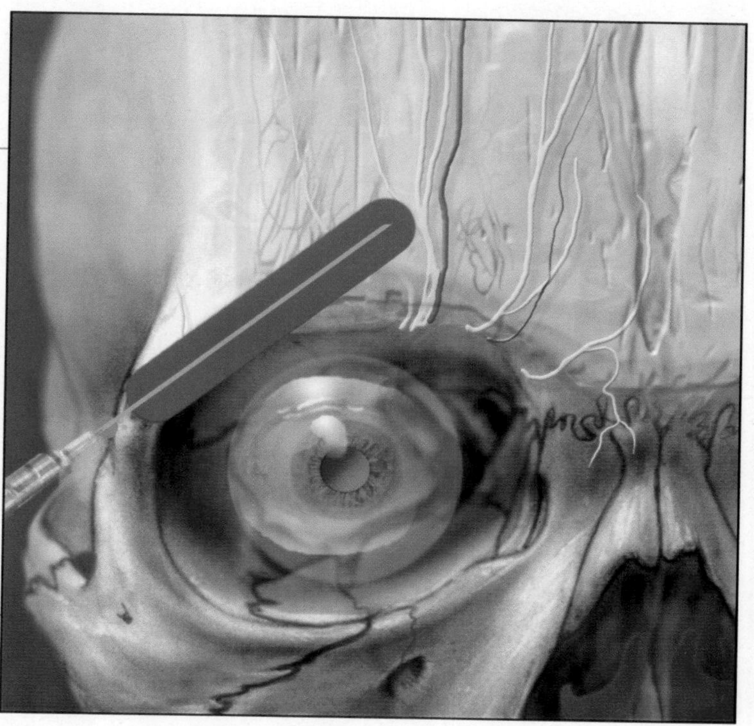

Figure 8.25

The lacrimal nerve, smallest branch off the ophthalmic branch of cranial nerve V, courses along the superior belly of the lateral rectus accompanied by the similarly named artery. In it are parasympathetic fibers for the lacrimal gland, and some sensory branches continue as noted. I have not personally seen this nerve, but removal of retro-orbicularis oculi fat (ROOF) often leaves the lateral brow numb.

The lacrimal nerve probably curls around the superolateral rim to supply the lateral eyebrow and upper lid area. Injection along the superolateral rim will block this nerve.

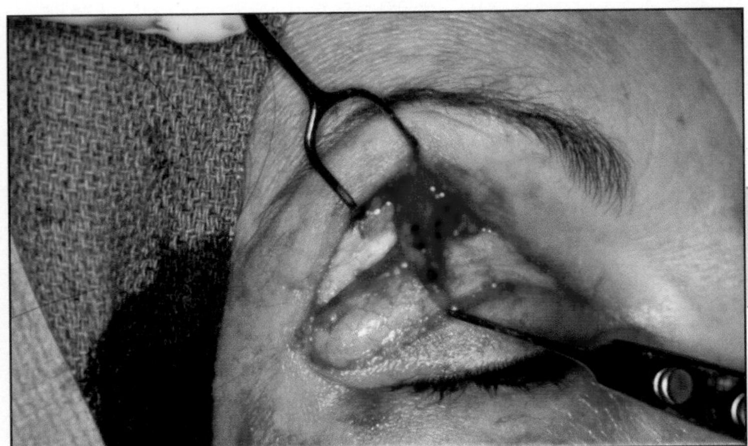

Figure 8.26

Removal of ROOF may yield some numbness of the lateral brow region. The forceps is grasping submuscular fat overlying the superolateral rim.

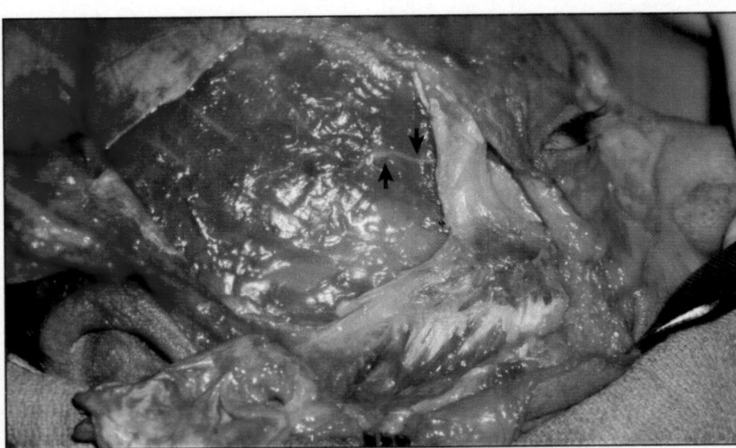

Figure 8.27

The arrows depict the zygomaticotemporal nerve, which exits through a hole behind the lateral rim about at canthal level, and often below. This nerve, seen here with the deep temporal fascia removed, then turns vertically to supply the lateral canthal and temporal region.

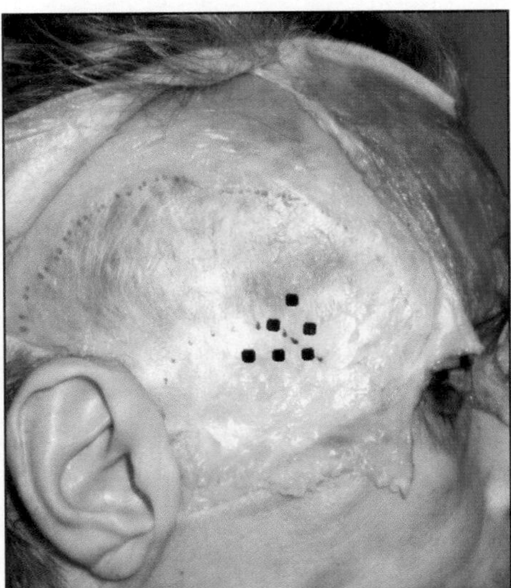

Figure 8.28

The black squares denote where the nerves would be perpendicular to the skin on exit through the fascia toward the skin.

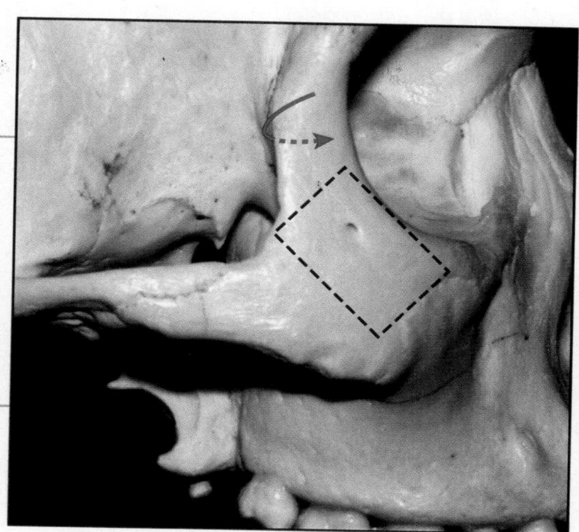

Figure 8.29

The *zygomaticotemporal* nerve exits a foramen near the level of the lateral canthus behind the rim (*red arrow*); the injection must follow the bone along the back of the rim or under the fascia (DTF) just behind the rim. The zygomaticofacial nerve exits one or more foramina in the area noted by dotted lines.

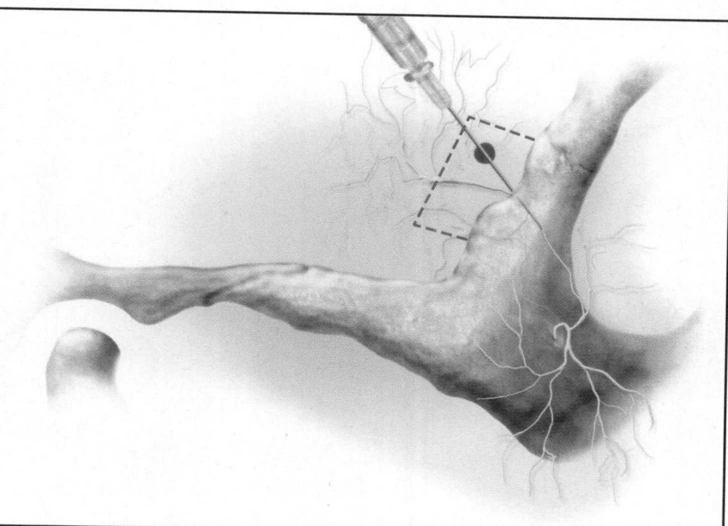

Figure 8.30

Zygomaticotemporal (z-t) block. This picture is not exact. I prefer to use an entrance point a bit higher and farther back than shown. This allows the needle to follow the back wall of the rim more easily. As noted the block may also be done subfascial in the dotted area.

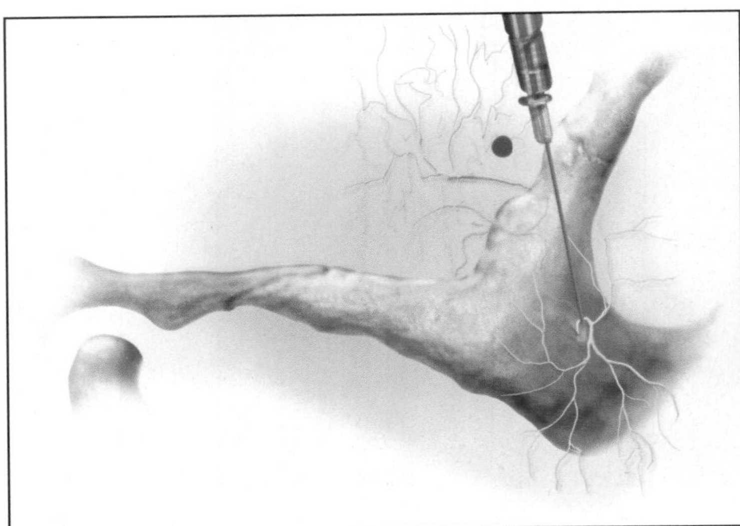

A

Figure 8.31A

The zygomaticofacial nerve(s) always exit below the lateral orbital retaining ligaments. Dropping 1 to 2 mL of local anesthetic lateral to and below the junction of inferior and lateral rim, just on the periosteum, will work well. An inverted triangular region will be blocked.

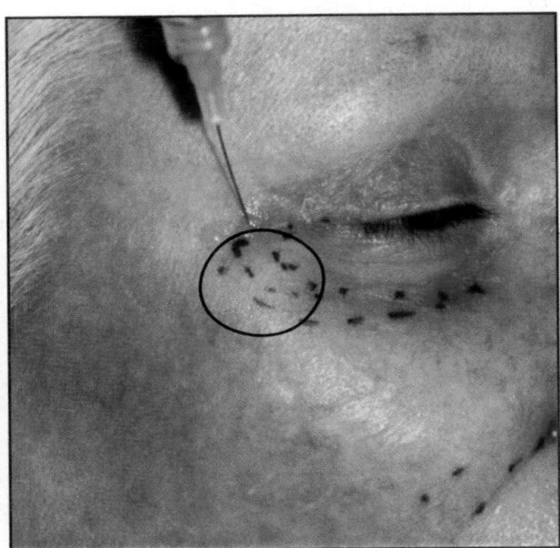

B

Figure 8.31B

Block in vivo.

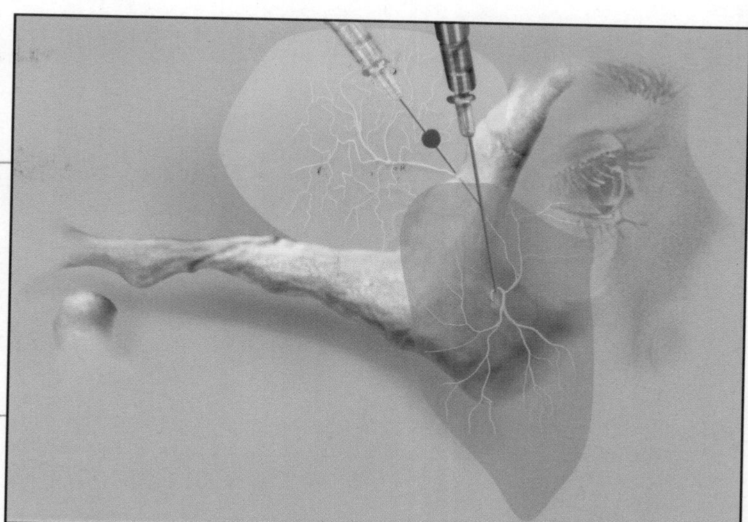

Figure 8.32

Any block may work on a larger or smaller area than expected. For example, the infraorbital and zygomaticofacial nerves meet to cover the entire lower eyelid. That area of overlap varies. This illustration shows the areas of the zygomaticotemporal (*yellow*) and zygomaticofacial (*gray*) nerves.

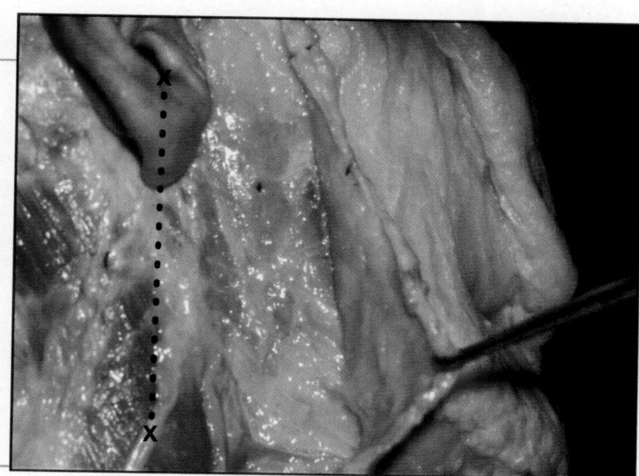

Figure 8.33

The distance from the lower external acoustic meatus (EAC) to where the great auricular nerve lies on the midsternocleidomastoid is about 6.5 cm. The external jugular (visible) is always about 1 cm closer anterior to the nerve at that point. This nerve supplies sensation to an area behind the ear at least halfway up the lobule and to a large area in front of the ear at the region of the angle of the mandible. Cervical plexus nerves exit at the front of the muscle to supply the neck.

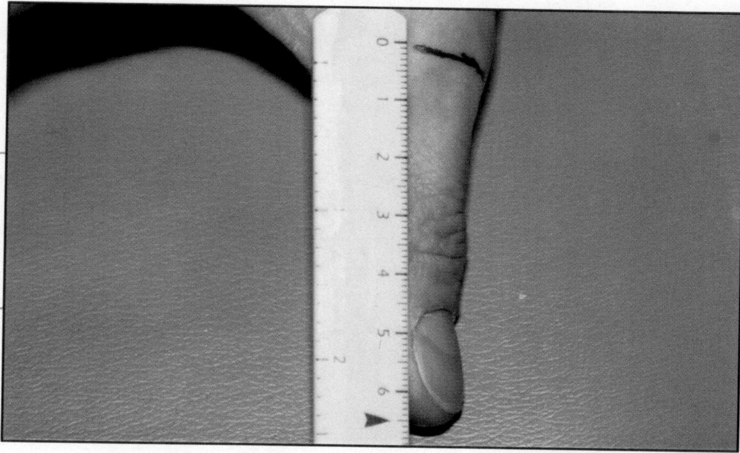

Figure 8.34

On my thumb, this is a perfect 6.5 cm; for others, it may be the length of the little finger. Find your own reference points or use a ruler for 6.5 cm.

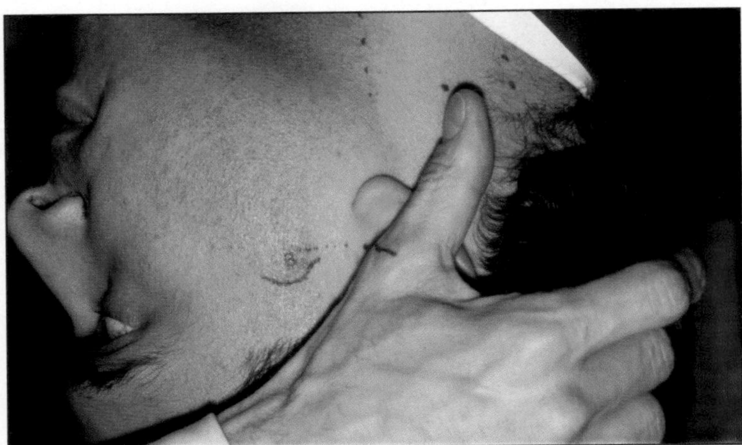

Figure 8.35

A dot is placed at 6.5 cm, and the injection goes to *fascia* in this region. About 2 to 3 mL of local anesthetic fanned in this area will work right on the muscle. The picture is upside down as I am usually at the head of the table to do this block.

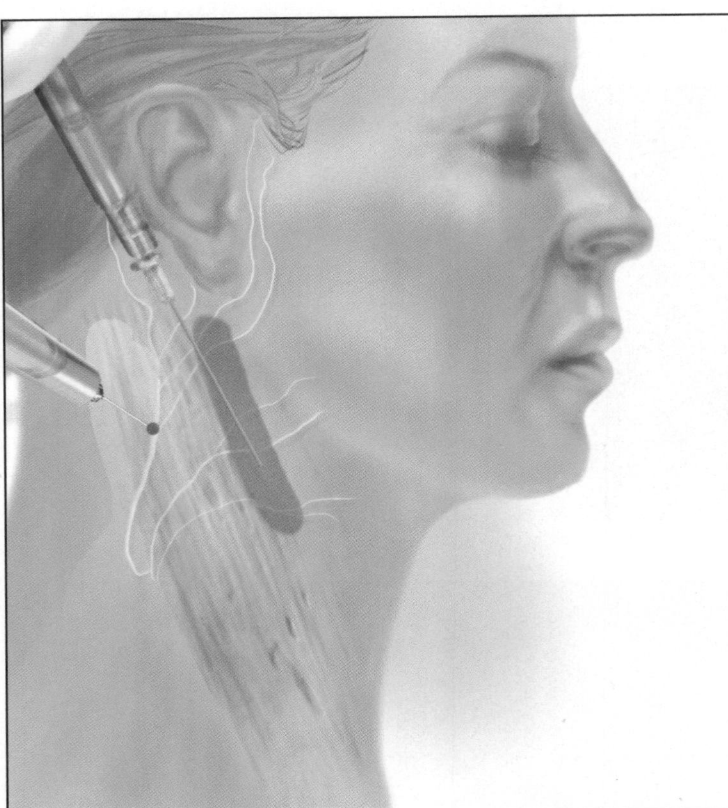

Figure 8.36

Next, the syringe is placed deeply along the anterior sternocleidomastoid (SCM) edge, and the injection is done in one to two passes on the way out to affect the upper neck and lower jaw line.

Figure 8.37

The space between the coronoid process (crow's beak) and the condyle is the U-shaped sigmoid notch. In thinner people, you can palpate it easily as your finger goes into a depression below the arch and 1 in. in front of the lower tragus. Below the skin, the fascia and masseter muscle may vary greatly in size, and in big-jowled persons the notch may be less easily palpable.

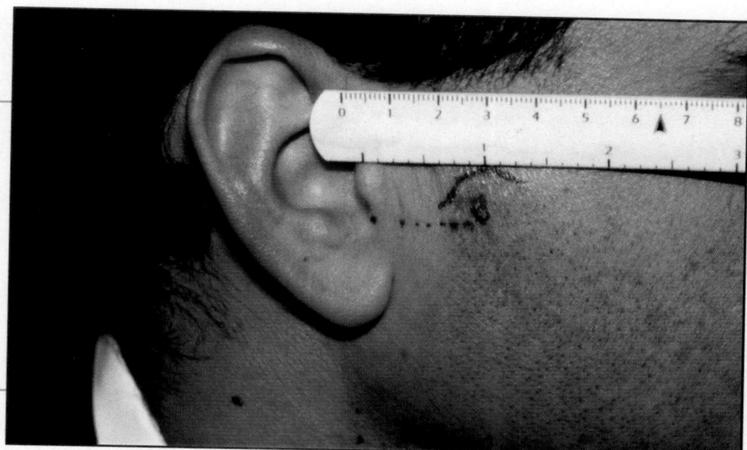

Figure 8.38A

Starting with a 25- or 27-gauge, 1½-in. needle, local anesthetic is injected in the skin and the needle is passed inward through the masseter to make sure you are going through the notch. The notch can be enlarged if the patient opens the teeth about a centimeter. Then, with a 22-gauge spinal needle, set the mobile plastic guard at about 4.5 cm and go through the numb area to hit the pterygoid plate (lateral) –x. (See below) The needle is then withdrawn and directed back about 1 cm at the same distance at which the plate was hit. After aspiration, inject 4–5 cc.

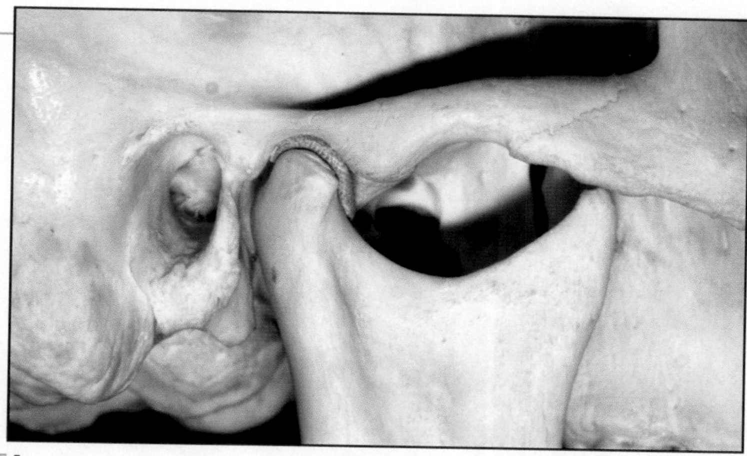

A

Figure 8.38B

With a small amount of practice, you will be able to do this with one pass directed slightly posteriorly. Remember, because the internal maxillary artery and many veins are in the area, aspirate prior to injection to avoid intravascular injections, which usually will lead to palpitations because of adrenalin.

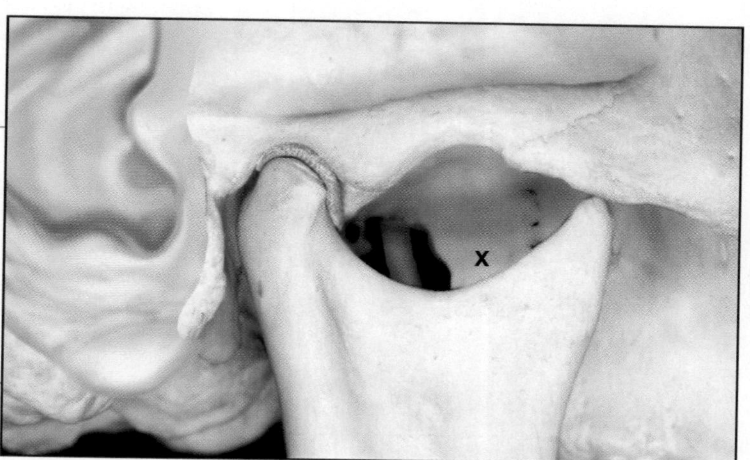

B

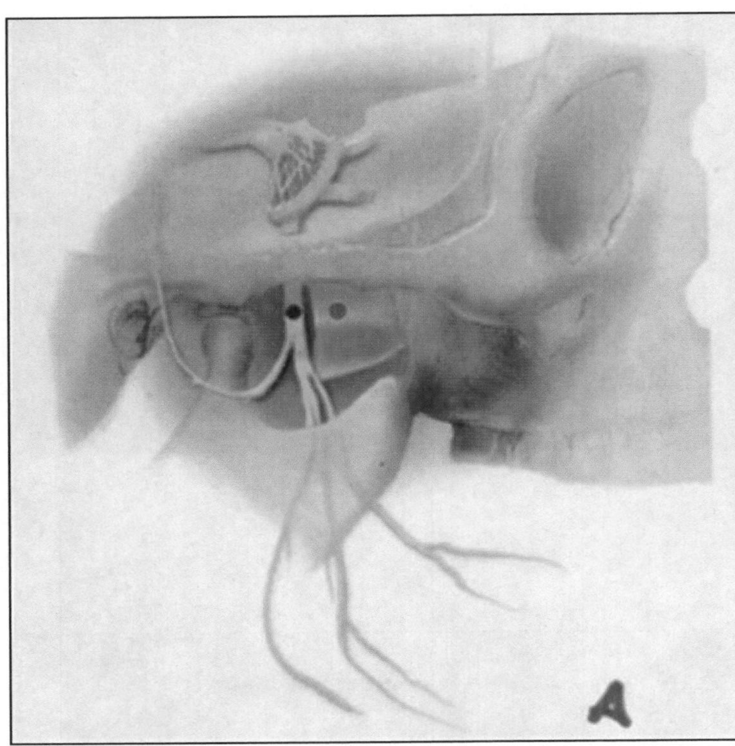

Figure 8.39

Once the pterygoid plate is hit (*red*), set the guard at that point, withdraw the 22-gauge spinal needle almost to the skin, and aim slightly back to the same depth. Then, aspirate and inject 4 to 5 mL. The buccal nerve for the cheek and the auriculotemporal nerve for the scalp will be anesthetized, as will the other branches of cranial nerve V_3. Note the effect of slight incisal opening.

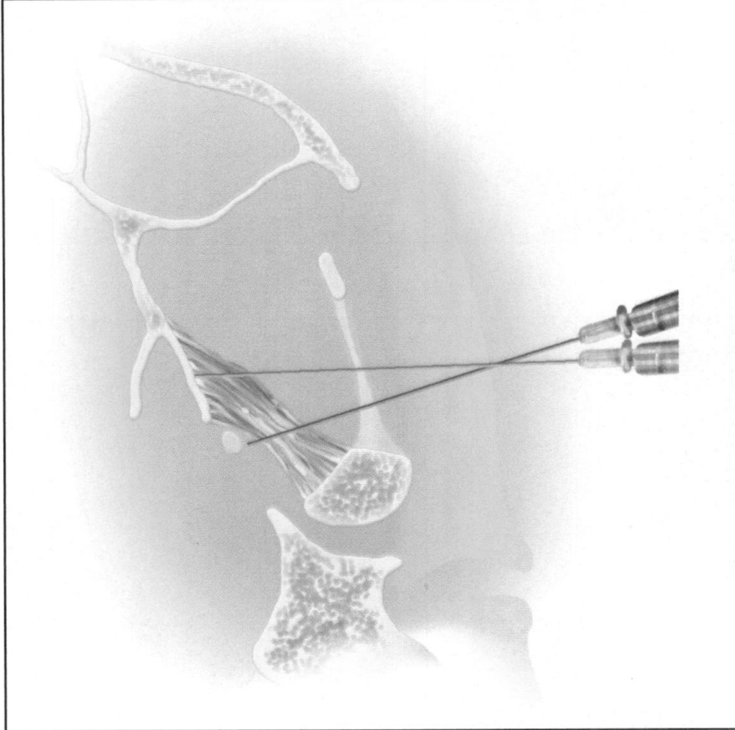

Figure 8.40

A cross-sectional view shows the initial pass of the red needle and then the more posteriorly directed blue needle hitting the nerve behind the lateral pterygoid muscle.

The cutaneous branches of V_3 supply the chin (via the inferior alveolar/mental), the skin over the lateral mandible and the fleshy cheek, and an area extending upward in front of the ear and including much of the temporal region.

Actually, regarding the ear, some of the tragus, anterior helical crus, and upper EAC may be affected. The buccal nerve will also affect the mucosa inside the cheek.